Surgical Atlas of Perforator Flaps

Chunlin Hou • Shimin Chang
Jian Lin • Dajiang Song

Surgical Atlas of Perforator Flaps

A Microsurgical Dissection Technique

Springer

Chunlin Hou
Department of Orthopedic Surgery
Changzheng Hospital
Second Military Medical University
Shanghai
China

Jian Lin
Department of Microsurgery
Xinhu Hospital
Shanghai Jiao Tong University
Shanghai
China

Shimin Chang
Department of Orthopedic Surgery
Yangpu Hospital
Tongji University School of Medicine
Shanghai
China

Dajiang Song
Department of Orthopedic Surgery
Changzheng Hospital
Second Military Medical University
Shanghai
China

ISBN 978-94-017-9833-4 ISBN 978-94-017-9834-1 (eBook)
DOI 10.1007/978-94-017-9834-1

Library of Congress Control Number: 2015938238

Springer Dordrecht Heidelberg New York London

Printed on acid-free paper

Springer Science+Business Media B.V. Dordrecht is part of Springer Science+Business Media (www.springer.com)

Contents

A Brief History of Perforator Flaps

1

Flap, or surgical flap in MeSH (Medical Subject Headings), is defined as a viable tissue block that has its own circulatory system and can survive independently by itself. If the tissue block has cutaneous tissue, it is called skin flap or cutaneous flap. In surgery, flaps are used to repair wound, to reconstruct function, and to restore esthetic appearance.

1.1 An Overview of the Development of Flaps

The reliability of any type of surgical flaps depends on the maintenance of an adequate blood circulation [1–4]. The history of skin flaps is a reflection of the study to better understand the anatomy of their vascular supply (Table 1.1). The early random-pattern flaps were constrained by rigorous length-to-width ratios to ensure viability. In 1970, Milton by experimental studies revealed that flap survival was dependent in fact on the intrinsic blood supply, not the strict mathematical length-to-breadth ratio. The axial-pattern flap concept was introduced by McGregor and Jackson in 1972, in their description of the groin flap. In 1970s, musculocutaneous flaps that were introduced by Ger and Orticochea rapidly became popular because of their reliability and wide arcs of rotation. In 1981, Pontén reported concept of fasciocutaneous flaps that greater length-to-width ratios could be achieved in flaps from the lower leg if the deep fascia was included. The anatomical basis for these fasciocutaneous flaps, which relied on the "fascial plexus" between the deep fascia and subdermal plexus, was later described by Haertsch, and Cormack and Lamberty. In 1987, following reappraisal of the early works of Manchot and Salmon, Taylor and Palmer published their work defining the vascular territories of source arteries, which they termed angiosomes.

China has pioneered in microsurgery since the first successful distal forearm replantation in 1963 by Dr. Zhong-Wei Chen, the first successful second toe-to-thumb transplantation in 1966 by Drs. Dong-Yue Yang and Yu-Dong Gu, the third free flap (lower abdomen flap nourished by superficial epigastric artery and vein) transfer in the world in 1973 also by Drs. Yang and Gu, and the first neurovascular pectoralis major (abdomen part) free transfer in 1973 by Dr. Zhong-Wei Chen's group. Microsurgical anatomy in new flap development was also extensively carried out in China. Professor Shi-Zhen Zhong, an anatomist, established an institute for microsurgical anatomy in Guangzhou and built a bridge between clinical microsurgery practice and basic microsurgical anatomy. Generally speaking, the major contributions to flap development by Chinese can be classified into three categories: (1) the main trunk artery flaps, (2) the reverse-flow island flaps with a distal main artery and venae comitantes, and (3) septocutaneous flaps avoid the sacrifice of the main artery trunk. These were fully represented in two flap donor sites: the radial forearm flap (Chinese flap) and the anterolateral thigh (ALT) flap [7, 8].

C. Hou et al., *Surgical Atlas of Perforator Flaps: A Microsurgical Dissection Technique*,
DOI 10.1007/978-94-017-9834-1_1, © Springer Science+Business Media Dordrecht 2015

Table 1.1 An overview of flap history

Time publication	Author(s)	Items
1956	Littler	Digital neurovascular island flap
1970	Milton	Experiment of length-to-width ratio
1972	McGregor, Morgan	Groin flap
1973	McGregor	Axial- and random-pattern flaps
1977	McCraw	Musculocutaneous flap
1981	Mathes, Nahai	Classification of vascular anatomy of muscles
1981	Yang	Radial forearm flap
1981	Ponten	Fasciocutaneous flap
1981	Nakayama	Arterialized venous flap
1982	Zhong	Anatomy of septocutaneous vessels
1982	Wang, Lu	Reverse-flow island flap
1984	Xu, Song	Anterolateral thigh flap
1984	Cormack, Lamberty	Classification of fasciocutaneous flap
1987	Taylor	Angiosomes
1989	Koshima	Perforator flap
1992	Bertelli, Masquelet	Neurocutaneous flap

1.2 An Overview of Perforator Flaps

Perforator flaps represent the latest descendant in a line of evolution that began with the random-pattern flap, musculocutaneous flap, and fasciocutaneous flap (Table 1.2). In surgery, the perforator flap era began in 1989, when Koshima and Soeda [5] described an inferior epigastric artery skin flap without rectus abdominis muscle for reconstruction of floor-of-the-mouth and groin defects, noting that a large flap without muscle could survive on a single muscle perforator. Kroll and Rosenfield suggested that perforator flaps combine the reliable blood supply of musculocutaneous flaps with the reduced donor-site morbidity of a skin flap. The reduced donor-site morbidity often leads to faster recovery and reduced postoperative pain. Perforator flaps have the additional advantages that they can be tailored to accurately reconstruct the defect, including flap thinning for resurfacing shallow defects; there is freedom of orientation of the pedicle; and a longer pedicle is harvested than with the parent musculocutaneous flap. There is hyperperfusion of the skin paddle, which may allow the capture of the adjacent two angiosomes, explaining how a single perforator can survive such a large flap area.

Originally, the concept of perforator flaps is attributed to musculocutaneous perforators only. However, extensive clinical practice had broadened the concept to contain all kinds of cutaneous perforators. Generally, two kinds of perforators existed: musculocutaneous (MC) and septocutaneous (SC).

In 1983, Professor Zhong's group proposed the concept of septocutaneous flaps, which was supplied by the septocutaneous branch (now called septocutaneous perforator), avoiding the sacrifice of major trunk artery. This is the first septocutaneous concept, in Chinese [6] (Fig. 1.1).

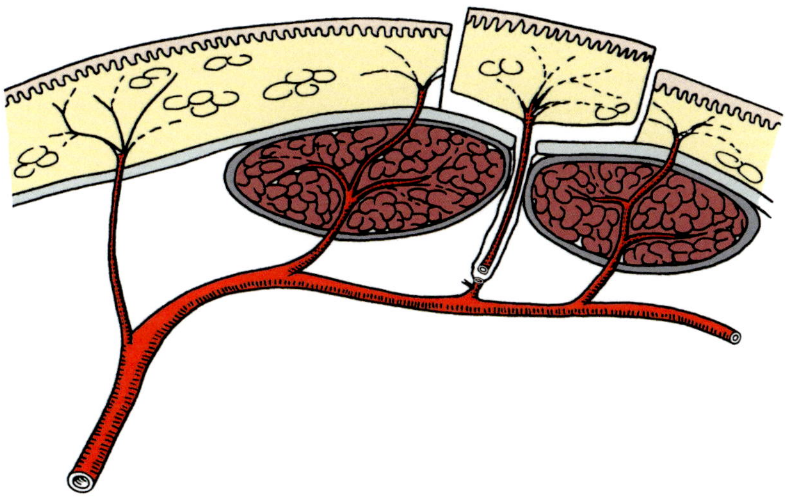

Fig. 1.1 Septocutaneous vessels (First proposed by Prof. Shi-Zhen Zhong in 1983)

Table 1.2 A brief history of perforator flaps

Time publication	Author(s)	Items
1889	Manchot	Skin vascular territory
1936	Salmon	The anatomic concept of perforator
1981	Mathes, Nahai	Anatomic classification of muscle vessels
1983	Zhong	Anatomy of septocutaneous vessel
1988	Kroll	Perforator-based flap
1989	Koshima	The concept of perforator flap

References

1. Strauch B, Vasconz LO, Hall-Findlay E, Lee BT. Grabb's encyclopedia of flaps. 3rd ed. New York: Wolter Kluwer Lippincott Williams & Wilkins; 2009.
2. Cormack GG, Lamberty BGH. The arterial anatomy of skin flaps. 2nd ed. Edinburgh: Churchill Livingstone; 1994. p. 255–7.
3. Ponten B. The fasciocutaneous flap: its use in soft tissue defects of the lower leg. Br J Plast Surg. 1981; 34:215–20.
4. Masquelet AC, Romana MC, Wolf G. Skin island flaps supplied by the vascular axis of the sensitive superficial nerve: anatomic study and clinical experience in the leg. Plast Reconstr Surg. 1992;89:1115–21.
5. Koshima I, Soeda S. Inferior epigastric artery skin flaps without rectus abdominis muscle. Br J Plast Surg. 1989;42:645–8.
6. Zhong SZ, Sun B, Liu MZ, Xu DC. Anatomical study of septocutaneous vessels [in Chinese]. Chin J Surg (ZhonghuaWai Ke Za Zhi). 1983;21:596–8.
7. Hou CL, Chang SM. History of Chinese society and state of practice in China. Microsurgery. 2008;28(1):2–3.
8. Chang SM, Hou CL, Xu DC. An overview of skin flap surgery in the mainland China: 20 years' achievements (1981 to 2000). J Reconstr Microsurg. 2009;25(6):361–7.

2 Anatomy, Classification, and Nomenclature

2.1 Perforator Vessel Types

There are two types of perforating vessels to the skin [1, 2]. They originate from the deep source artery, passing directly to the overlying fascia and skin, from a cavity or fissure that lacks deep fascia (direct cutaneous artery, e.g., axillary fossa, cubital fossa, oval fossa, and popliteal fossa) or the septum, or passing some tissue structures (mostly muscles) and then indirectly to the skin (Fig. 2.1).

1. Musculocutaneous perforators: this type of perforator is the cutaneous vessel after penetrating underlying muscle. Through intramuscular dissection, longer vascular pedicle can be obtained.
2. Septocutaneous perforators: this type of perforator is the cutaneous vessel after piercing the fascial septum between muscles. Through intraseptal dissection, the perforator can be traced to its deep origin from the source artery (Fig. 2.2).

C. Hou et al., *Surgical Atlas of Perforator Flaps: A Microsurgical Dissection Technique*,
DOI 10.1007/978-94-017-9834-1_2,

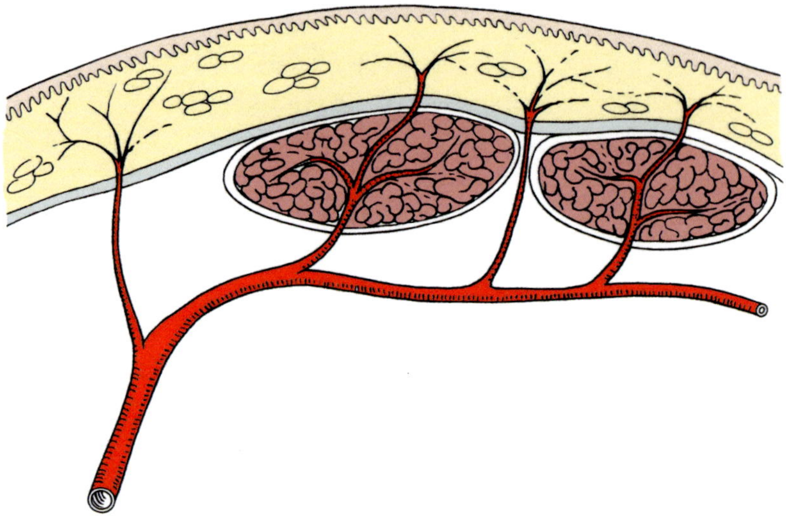

Fig. 2.1 Types of perforating vessels to the skin

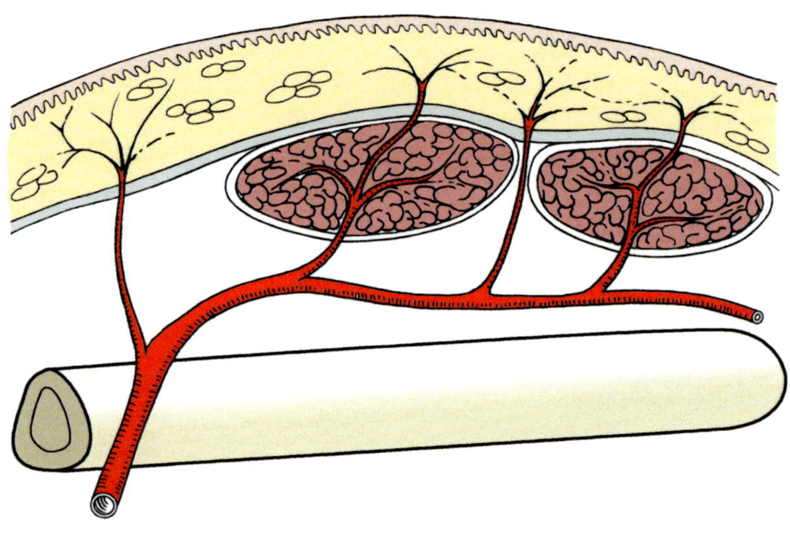

Fig. 2.2 The perforator can be traced to its deep origin from the source artery

2.2 Vascular Plexus of the Integument

There are five layers of vascular plexus in the integument, from deep to surface; it is subfascial, suprafascial, adiposal, subdermal, and dermal. If some specific structures exist in the subcutaneous tissue, for example, superficial sensitive nerve and/or subcutaneous vein, there are perineural and/or perivenous plexus (Fig. 2.3).

Three vascular plexus of integument are rich and abundant – suprafascial plexus, perineural and perivenous plexus, and subdermal plexus – and they are corresponding to the concept of fasciocutaneous flap, neurocutaneous flap, and thinned flap, respectively [3-6].

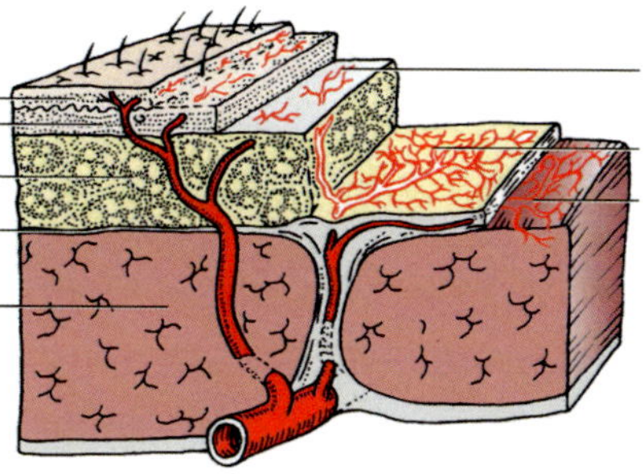

Fig. 2.3 Vascular plexuses of the integument

2.3 Classification of Perforator Flaps

From the point of vascular anatomy, there are two types of perforator flaps, musculocutaneous perforator flap and septocutaneous perforator flap.

Perforator flaps can also be classified by its tissue composition (flap constitutes), transferring mode (pedicled or free), contiguity (local or distant), and other characteristics [7, 8] (Table 2.1).

Table 2.1 Types of perforator flaps

Basic type	Isolated perforator pedicle nourishing a skin island	Perforator flap (adipocutaneous)
		Perforator fasciocutaneous flap
		Perforator-adipofascial flap
		Perforator subcutaneous-fat flap
		Perforator thinned flap
		Perforator neurocutaneous flap
Perforator extended	Perforator-plus-adipofascial pedicle	Perforator-adipofascial flap
		Perforator-adipofascial neurocutaneous flap
Perforator combined	Source artery and perforator tree	Perforator conjoint flap (Siamese)
		Perforator chimeric flap
		Perforator flow-through flap

2.4 Nomenclature of Perforator Flaps

There have been many debates about the concept and terminology of perforator flaps, until 2001 when a group of experts reach a consensus in Belgian [9] (Table 2.2).

2.4.1 A New Nomenclature by Chinese Microsurgery Society

The Gent consensus published in 2003 on perforator flap terminology is still the keystone and guideline for scientific communications. However, some modifications must be made to accommodate the rapid and prosperous progress, both in clinical applications and basic investigations [11, 12]. Since 2005, the Chinese microsurgery society has held panels to discuss perforator flaps every year and has reached consensus on definition and nomenclature. The Chinese terminology of perforator flaps is based primarily to the six definitions in the Gent consensus [3], but with some modifications (Table 2.3). This may be relatively broad and may contain various variants in clinical applications.

Table 2.2 The "Gent" consensus on perforator flap terminology (Blondeel [9])

Definition 1	A perforator flap is a flap consisting of skin and/or subcutaneous fat. The vessels that supply blood to the flap are isolated perforator(s). These perforators may pass either through or in between the deep tissues (mostly muscle)
Definition 2	A muscle perforator is a blood vessel that traverses through muscle to supply the overlying skin
Definition 3	A septal perforator is a blood vessel that traverses only through septum to supply the overlying skin
Definition 4	A flap that is vascularized by a muscle perforator is called a muscle perforator flap
Definition 5	A flap vascularized by a septal perforator is called a septal perforator flap
Definition 6	A perforator flap should be named after the nutrient artery or vessels and not after the underlying muscle. If there is a potential to harvest multiple perforator flaps from one vessel, the name of each flap should be based on its anatomical region or muscle

Table 2.3 Chinese version of perforator flap definition and nomenclature

Definition	All flaps isolated on a set of perforator vessels (artery and vein, one or several) can be defined as perforator flaps. It is an axial-pattern flap, nourished directly by tiny perforator vessels (intraseptal or intramuscular) that must be identified or isolated during operative microdissection	Perforator flaps are defined from the point of feeding vessels, regardless of flap tissue component, i.e., a perforator flap can be adipocutaneous, fasciocutaneous, or neurocutaneous and adiposal, adipofascial, or fascial, etc.
Application	Perforator flaps can be clinically used in fashions such as free (microvascular anastomosis), pedicled (pure perforator, or perforator-plus), combined (conjoint, chimeric, flow-through) or vascular augmented (supercharged, turbocharged, or superdrainaged), and so on	
Nomenclature	A perforator flap should be named preferably after the nutrient artery or vessels and not after the underlying muscle. If there is a potential to harvest multiple perforator flaps from one vessel, the name of each perforator flap should be based on its anatomical region and the proximal vessel or muscle and proximal vessel (Figs. 2.4 and 2.5)	Differentiation at the vascular level Medial sural artery (*with*) perforator flap means at least a segment of medial sural artery is harvested and included in the pedicle Medial sural artery (*without*) perforator flap means the flap is a true perforator flap and no deep source vessel is harvested

(continued)

Table 2.3 (continued)

Usage	Two versions of nomenclature can be used practically	For oral communication or in the title of a paper, concise version should be used, usually named as "proximal vessel + perforator flap," "anatomical region + perforator flap," or "muscle + perforator flap." For introducing new perforator vessels or anatomical variations, or in the text and patient table of a paper, precise version should be used, such as the Sinna [10] method with a series of abbreviations

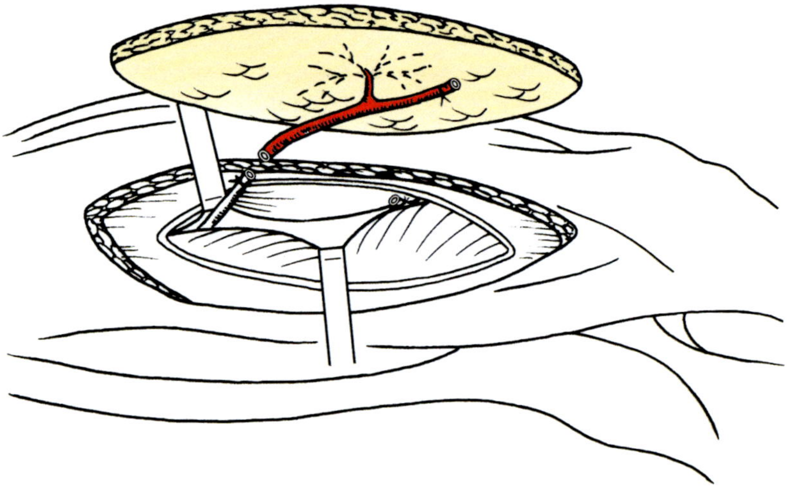

Fig. 2.4 Perforator flap with source vessel

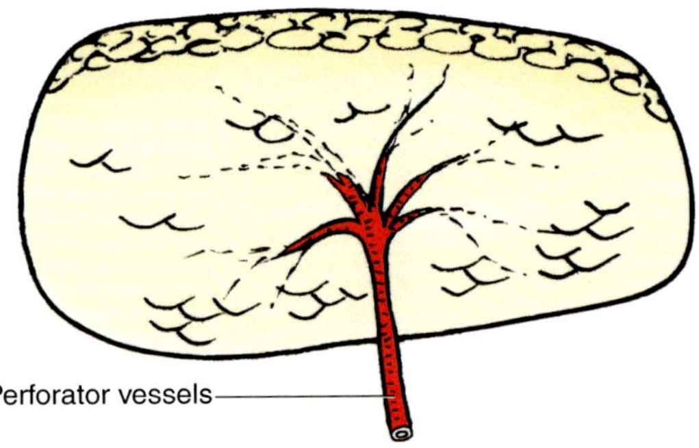

Fig. 2.5 Perforator flap without source vessel, true perforator

References

1. Cormack GG, Lamberty BGH. The arterial anatomy of skin flaps. 2nd ed. Edinburgh: Churchill Livingstone; 1994.
2. Zhong SZ, Sun B, Liu MZ, Xu DC. Anatomical study of septocutaneous vessels [in Chinese]. Chin J Surg (Zhonghua Wai Ke Za Zhi). 1983;21:596–8.
3. Carriquiry CE, Costa MA, Vasconez LO. The anatomic study of the septocutaneous vessels of the leg. Plast Reconstr Surg. 1985;76:354–61.
4. Pignatti M, Ogawa R, Hallock GG, et al. The "Tokyo" consensus on propeller flaps. Plast Reconstr Surg. 2011;127:716–22.
5. Tang ML, Mao YH, Almutairi K, et al. Three-dimensional analysis of perforators of the posterior leg. Plast Reconstr Surg. 2009;123:1729–38.
6. Taylor GI, Pan WR. Angiosomes of the leg: anatomic study and clinical implications. Plast Reconstr Surg. 1998;102:599–616.
7. Koshima I, Soeda S. Inferior epigastric artery skin flaps without rectus abdominis muscle. Br J Plast Surg. 1989;42:645–8.
8. Saint-Cyr M, Schaverien MV, Rohrich RJ. Perforator flaps: history, controversies, physiology, anatomy, and use in reconstruction. Plast Reconstr Surg. 2009;123:132e–45.
9. Blondeel PN, Van Landuyt KH, Monstrey SJ, Hamdi M, Matton GE, Allen RJ, et al. The "Gent" consensus on perforator flap terminology: preliminary definitions. Plast Reconstr Surg. 2003;112:1378–83.
10. Sinna R, Boloorchi A, Mahajan AL, Qassemyar Q, Robbe M. What should define a "perforator flap"? Plast Reconstr Surg. 2010;126:2258–63.
11. Hallock GG. The complete nomenclature for combined perforator flaps. Plast Reconstr Surg. 2011;127:1720–9.
12. Taylor GI, Rozen WM, Whitaker IS. Establishing a perforator flap nomenclature based on anatomical principles. Plast Reconstr Surg. 2012;129:877e–9.

3 Intraoperative Techniques in Perforator Dissection

In a selected donor site, raising a perforator flap entails: (1) localization of skin perforators using the handheld Doppler and (2) raising the flap by performing retrograde dissection from the perforator to the source vessel until a sufficient pedicle length and size has been achieved, regardless of the origin of the harvested vessel. This manner of flap elevation was firstly introduced by Wei and coauthors in 2004 and termed as free-style concept [1]. As a result of this concept, any skin paddle based on a substantially sized perforator, localized by an audible Doppler signal, can be potentially harvested. With a substantial number of available perforators in the body, this approach certainly increases the surgeon's degree of freedom in terms of reconstructive options [2].

3.1 Surgical Technique

1. The first step in performing a free-style perforator flap is locating sizable perforators in the selected region of the body. Handheld Doppler ultrasonography has been shown to be an accurate method of locating and mapping these cutaneous vessels. The operator carefully notes the quality of the Doppler sound detected with particular attention given to the location of loud, high-pitched, and pulsatile signals. The vessels with more prominent sounds are marked with a larger dot and selected as the vessel that is intended to dissect. The flap is then designed centered on these perforators.
2. Dissection is performed under loupe magnification (2.5–3.5×). Only one border of the proposed design should be incised initially for exploration. This affords the flexibility to alter the flap design should this be necessary based on intraoperative findings.
3. The flaps were dissected in the suprafascial plane to minimize donor-site morbidity by preserving fascia and cutaneous nerve that run immediately above the fascia. It is important to maintain meticulous hemostasis as excessive bleeding and subsequent staining of the tissues interferes with clear visualization and accurate identification of small vessels.
4. After sizable cutaneous vessels are found, the deep fascia is cut to start mobilizing the vessels. This may entail intramuscular dissection for musculocutaneous perforators or may be relatively straightforward in the case of septocutaneous perforators. Retrograde mobilization of the vascular pedicle is continued until a sufficient length and/or size is achieved. Depending on the size of the perforators and the size of the flap that need to be harvested, the flap can be based on a single perforator or multiple perforators.
5. Once all these crucial surgical decisions have been made and flap dimensions and design confirmed, the flap is completely islanded and the pedicle divided. In general, the average size of a single perforator-based flap is 100–200 cm^2.
6. Because of the inherent unpredictability of pedicle size and length, the surgeon should

C. Hou et al., *Surgical Atlas of Perforator Flaps: A Microsurgical Dissection Technique*,
DOI 10.1007/978-94-017-9834-1_3, © Springer Science+Business Media Dordrecht 2015

Table 3.1 The six technical rules for surgical elevation of perforator flap

	Rules	Explanations
1.	Try to map the perforator preoperatively	Locate the perforator and estimate its size and branches, by anatomical data, handheld Doppler, color Duplex, CT angiography
2.	Try to identify the main perforator by making a limited exploratory incision on only one side	Leave the opportunity of backup plan during operation, for example, to conventional flap
3.	Preserve each perforator until you encounter a large one	Simple philosophy to enhance safety in the decision-making process
4.	Select the best perforator	Considering its size, concomitant vein, location, length, etc.
5.	Consider the easiest dissection	Intramuscular dissection is tedious; involvement with motor nerve branches increases complexity
6.	Transect perforators that will not be used after the entire pedicle is dissected	

always have a "backup" plan when attempting a free-style perforator flap. The first exploratory incision should be always performed to allow the opportunity of using of the "backup" flap. In the thigh, for example, if the mapped vessel is located in the medial thigh, the first incision should be along with the lateral margin over the skin paddle. The dissection should be from lateral to medial. If no suitable skin vessels are encountered, the dissection direction will be shifted toward the lateral side for the harvest of the "backup" ALT flap.

7. Critical to the success of harvesting a free-style perforator flap is the intramuscular perforator dissection. Gentle handling is important to prevent vasospasm that may be sometimes irreversible. These are very delicate flaps that need gentle handling in every stage from harvest to inset. Its pedicle consists of a small perforator that has been completely skeletonized during harvest and lacks a protective cuff of soft tissue around the site where the perforator enters the flap. These features make it particularly susceptible to kinking, compression, and even rupture during the inset.
8. The harvested perforator free flap is then transferred to the recipient site by vascular anastomosis.

There is a learning curve for every new procedure. Reading books and articles to get sufficient knowledge and follow standard steps can shorten the learning time, avoid mistakes, and prevent complications. The philosophy is forward step-by-step and leaves the opportunity of salvage with alternative flaps (Table 3.1).

References

1. Wei FC, Mardini S. Free-style free flap. Plast Reconstr Surg. 2004;114(4):910–6.
2. Chang CC, Wong CH, Wei FC. Free-style free flap. Injury. 2008;39 Suppl 3:S57–61.

Pedicled Perforator Flaps

4

Pedicled perforator flaps are also called local perforator flaps, or island perforator flaps. It combines the advantages of pedicled local flaps (good color and texture match, like-with-like reconstruction), pedicled regional flaps (up to 180° arc of rotation), pedicled distant flap (vascular reliable and larger size), and without microsurgical vascular anastomosis. For most small- to medium-sized defects, pedicled perforator flap allows linear closure of the donor site.

Theoretically, a flap can be designed and harvested based on any dominant and clinically relevant perforator. With over 300 perforators in the body, a large number of flaps can be theoretically harvested when an appropriate perforator is selected. The principle of free-style local perforator flaps can be used and applied to harvest pedicle perforator flaps for reconstruction of various head and neck, trunk, and extremity defects.

First of all, the perforators in the vicinity of the defect were localized by noninvasive methods, for example, Doppler, Duplex, angiography, or CTA, then the flap can be designed and elevated.

There are two types perforator-pedicled island flaps, V-Y advancement flaps and propeller flaps (Fig. 4.1). The distally pedicled version of perforator flaps is very useful for limb reparative and reconstructive surgery, especially for the distal extremities such as wrist-hand and foot-ankle region, which is the focused topic in this book.

4.1 Selection of Flap Movement Fashion

The most important factor to determine flap movement (advancement versus propeller) is the distance between the emerging point of the perforator and the proximal margin of the defect (perforator-defect distance). If an audible signal is recognized in Doppler only in close proximity to the defect (perforator-defect distance < defect diameter), the project of a V-Y advancement flap should be carefully evaluated, and a propeller flap movement should be chosen. On the other hand, if the perforators are detected at an intermediate distance from the defect (perforator-defect distance ≥ defect diameter), the application of the V-Y advancement model is recommended.

Generally speaking, V-Y advancement moves shorter distance than propeller rotation. V-Y advancement is more suitable for head-neck and trunk region and more suitable for myocutaneous perforators. Propeller movement is more suitable for limbs and septocutaneous perforators (Table 4.1).

C. Hou et al., *Surgical Atlas of Perforator Flaps: A Microsurgical Dissection Technique*,
DOI 10.1007/978-94-017-9834-1_4, © Springer Science+Business Media Dordrecht 2015

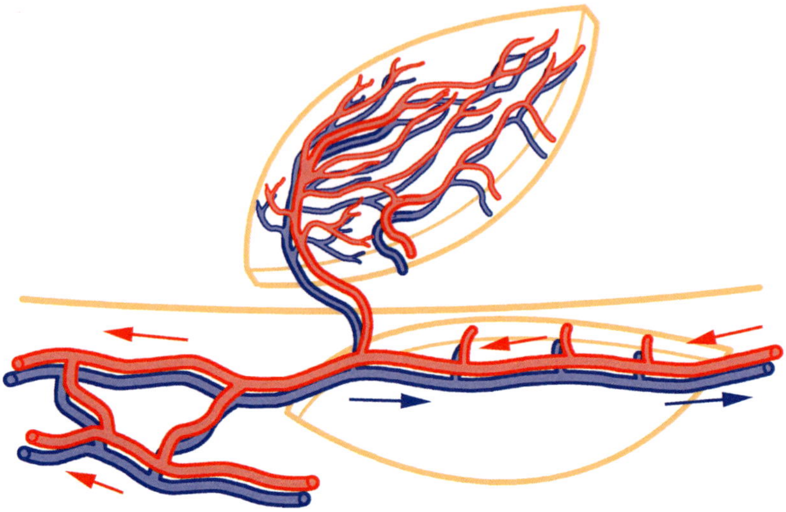

Fig. 4.1 Propeller flaps. Arterial perfusion direction (*red arrow*), venous drainage direction (*blue arrow*)

Table 4.1 Comparison of perforator-pedicled V-Y advancement flaps and propeller flaps

	V-Y advancement flaps	Propeller flaps
Pedicle movement	Advancement	Rotational
Range of movement	Small-medium	Wide
Flap size	Small-medium	Medium-large
No. of perforators	Multiple	Single
Possibility of converting to conventional "plan B" flap	Always maintained	Often maintained
Vascular safety	High	High, but unpredictable
Donor site	Primary closure	Skin graft for large defects

4.2 Perforator-Pedicled V-Y Advancement Flaps

The perforator-based version of the V-Y flap, being based on a fully dissected and isolated perforator, has a range of movement that is considerably wider than a classic V-Y flap. Its advantages are simplicity, speed of harvesting, and donor-site closure. Its drawbacks are limited movement, limited size, and transfer over the defect of the skin lying in close proximity to the wound.

A V-Y advancement flap is indicated for small, noncomplicated wounds when a good perforator can be isolated. The amount of tissue that can be transferred to cover the defect is limited by the perforator caliber and the amount of advancement by the perforator length. The skeletonized perforator is very sensitive to stretching and shearing, and it must not be pulled too much. The flap must be accurately planned before the skin is incised circumferentially. To avoid wound dehiscence, it must reach the recipient site without any tension. In contrast, the donor-site appearance is excellent, and after a few weeks, the scars may be almost invisible. The morbidity of the donor site is minimal.

4.2.1 Flap Design and Dimension

The length of the flap is planned to be 1.5–2 times the diameter of the defect in the direction of advancement, while the width is slightly larger than the width of the defect. These suggestions about length-to-width ratio reflect the geometrical constitution of the V-Y advancement model. Adherence to these general rules rather than to the classic length-to-width ratio is considered clinically safe and recommended in practice, as it is with ease for wound closure after the skin island advancement. The perforator V-Y advancement flaps are ideally centered on the axial perforator vessel and do not act as random-pattern flaps.

4.2.2 Exploratory Incision and Pedicle Dissection

Flaps are harvested with the aid of 2.5× loupe magnification. The exploratory incision is carried down to the deep fascia. On the extremities, a subfascial approach is preferred to expose and dissect the perforators. Once all the perforators have been identified, their position in the flap, their caliber, their pulsatility, and the presence of adequate venae comitantes are evaluated. The perforators chosen to obtain an advancement movement are carefully dissected for 2–3 cm by gently teasing the muscular fibers. Perforators are irrigated intermittently with 2 % lidocaine solution during flap dissection. Extensive intramuscular dissection is not mandatory and is recommended only when pedicle elongation is needed to improve flap advancement.

4.2.3 Skin Paddle Circumcision

A “cut-as-you-go” approach is applied to maximize vascular safety, while maintaining the opposite skin bridge until the end of dissection. If the presence of and good-quality perforator vessels have been confirmed, the skin paddle is redrawn according to the intraoperative findings and circumcised. If the flap reaches the defect without tension, all the dissected perforators are preserved, assuming that flaps based on more than one perforator could show a reduced incidence of vascular complications. The only limitation to the number of perforators to be included is the degree of flap advancement. In case of restricted movement, applying microclamps on minor perforators allows the surgeon to assess the dominance of the main perforator. After this surgical maneuver, if flap perfusion is confirmed, minor perforators are sacrificed to obtain further advancement.

In contrast, if the perforators are found to be of small diameter or of weak pulsatility at the end of dissection, a skin bridge is maintained on the other side to convert the flap to a perforator-plus model, which provides, despite of more difficult insetting, additional blood supply and improved venous outflow.

4.2.4 Factors Influencing Flap Advancement

Flap advancement is influenced by several factors:

1. Position of the skin island to the skin tension line.
2. Anatomical features of the perforator vessel. If possible, centering the flap on the main audible perforator is advisable, because eccentric pedicles may restrict flap advancement.
3. Types of perforator. Septocutaneous perforators, such as posterior tibial or peroneal artery perforators, despite good caliber, are found to be shorter and usually offer a lesser degree of advancement when compared with their medial sural artery counterparts, which is a myocutaneous perforator.
4. The direction of advancement in extremities. In case of distal flap movement, a lesser degree of advancement is expected (Fig. 4.2).

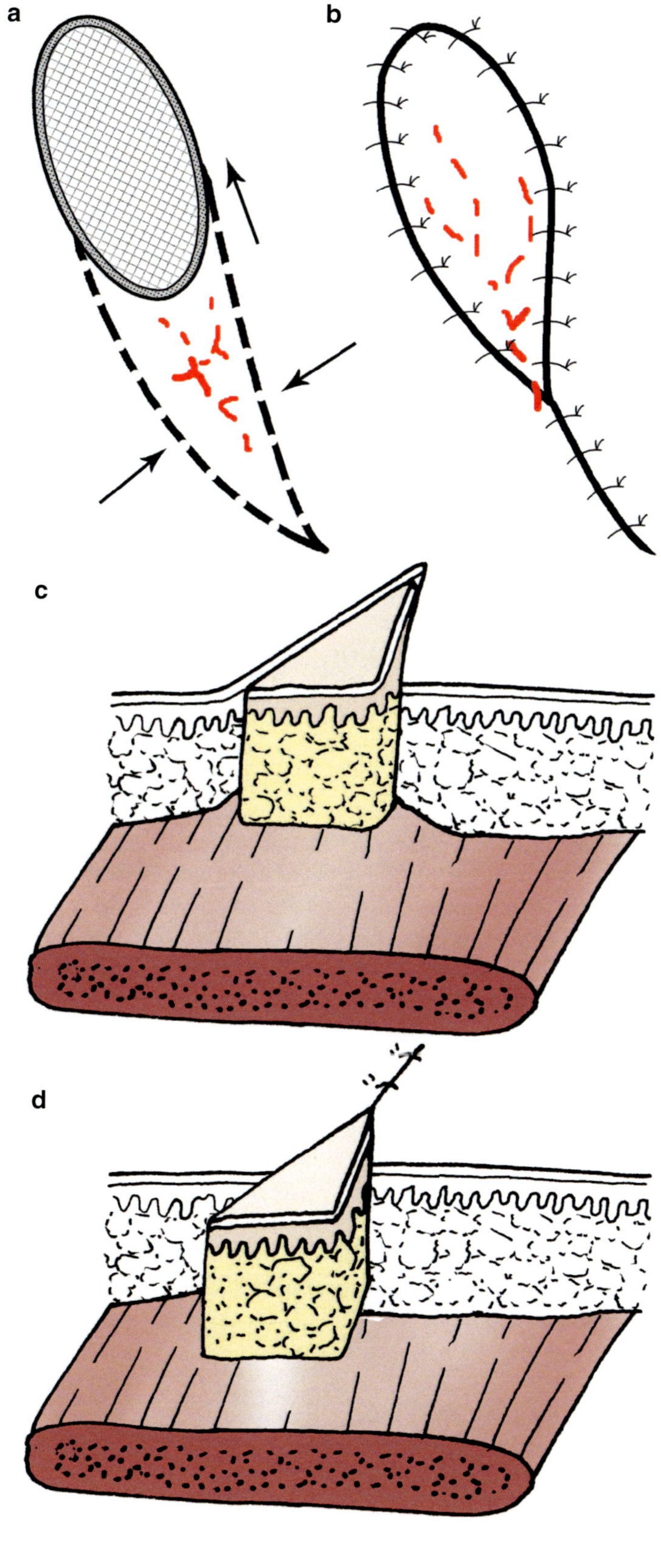

Fig. 4.2 Flap advancement. Preoperative Doppler investigation is performed to determine the entry point of the perforator. The incision was carried out according to the margin of the outlined flap. The flap is rotated to coover the defect, the donor site can be closed directly

4.3 Perforator-Pedicled Propeller Flaps

The peculiarity of the propeller flap is that its two blades are used to cover both the defect and, partially or totally, the donor site [1, 2]. These flaps may be raised as very long flaps not being limited by the rules of length-to-width ratios. A propeller flap can be long and narrow, but because the position of the pedicle is in the vicinity of the center of the flap, the actual dimensions of the flap nourished by the perforating pedicle are two flaps of approximately half the length of the total skin island (the two blades of the propeller) (Fig. 4.3).

4.3.1 Flap Design

The first thing to do is using a handheld Doppler ultrasound scanner to locate the most promising perforator artery around the defect. Then, a provisional flap design can be drawn. (1) The distance between the perforator and the distal edge of the defect is measured. This value is then transposed proximally, again measured from the perforator, and 1–2 cm is added. This forms the proximal limit of the flap. (2) The width of the flap needed to cover the defect is determined. The width of the defect is measured. This value is then used to determine the proximal flap width, adding 0.5–1 cm to allow for tissue contraction and to facilitate easy closure without tension. The elliptical skin island is designed so that the distance between the perforator and the distal portion of the flap is slightly longer than the distance between the perforator and the furthest part of the wound to prevent any risk of closing tension. It is important that the lateral dimensions of the flap, at the point where the perforator pedicle enters the flap, is equidistant in order that when the flap is eventually rotated around to fill the defect, there is no excessive sideway tension on the perforator during closure (Fig. 4.4).

4.3.2 Raising the Flap and Perforator Dissection [3–9]

A tourniquet is used and the leg is exsanguinated by elevation and compression of the popliteal artery for 1 min. This allows emptying of most of the blood from the leg but retains enough in the perforator vessels to allow for easier identification during exploration.

The perforator vessels are located through an exploratory initial incision. It is important for safety and easier assessment to make this incision long enough. The approach to the pedicle could be suprafascial or subfascial, with the latter being generally easier and less bloody. Unless you are already very experienced with raising perforator flaps, the subfascial approach is probably also safer as it is the surgical plane for flap elevation and allows easier visualization of the pedicle. With this initial incision, a number of potentially useful perforators can be found. A visual assessment of the perforators is then made to choose the best pedicle for the flap. This is based on its position, size, and whether there is any potential injury to the pedicle. In general, it would be wise to avoid a perforator that is within 1–2 cm from the wound (especially chronic wounds) unless there are no other suitable ones available. On the other hand, it is best not to choose a perforator too far away from the defect as this would make the flap unnecessarily long. When the decision is made, the perforator that is finally chosen for the flap may not necessarily be the one located preoperatively on Doppler ultrasound and on which the initial design of the flap is based. That is not a problem because the planning and raising of the flap should allow for flexibility of redesigning and adjustment of its dimension. With this approach, once you have decided that the pedicle chosen is the best in terms of its location, size, and suitability to sustain the flap, the design of the flap should be rechecked and if necessary adjusted. In particular, one should ensure that the proximal edge of the flap, when it is finally rotated into position, is capable of reaching the distal margin of the defect comfortably and would not place the pedicle under any tension.

Once that critical decision has been made about the perforator, careful dissection around the pedicle is taken. The pedicle should be cleared of all muscular side branches for at least 2 cm. If possible, try to clean the pedicle from its vessel of origin to the point where the pedicle penetrates the deep fascia of the flap. There should be a meticulous division of all the fascial strands that could potentially cause vascular embarrassment through kinking of the vessels. One should pay particular attention to those around the venae comitantes, since they are relatively low-pressure systems and are therefore more susceptible to compression once the flap is rotated into position. The safety of the flap is enhanced by such a radical dissection around the artery and venae comitantes. Obviously great care and gentleness should be employed during this crucial step of the operation. The use of magnification is important for this part of the dissection. A pair of 2.5× magnification loupes would be sufficient.

Once the pedicle is secured, raising the rest of the flap is quick and straightforward. Once the flap has been completely islanded, it should be left in its original position and the tourniquet released. It is important to allow it to perfuse and to allow the spasm of the vessels to relax, in its original position, for 10–15 min before the flap is rotated into the defect. Topical vasodilators, such as papaverine or verapamil, can be instilled around the pedicle at this point.

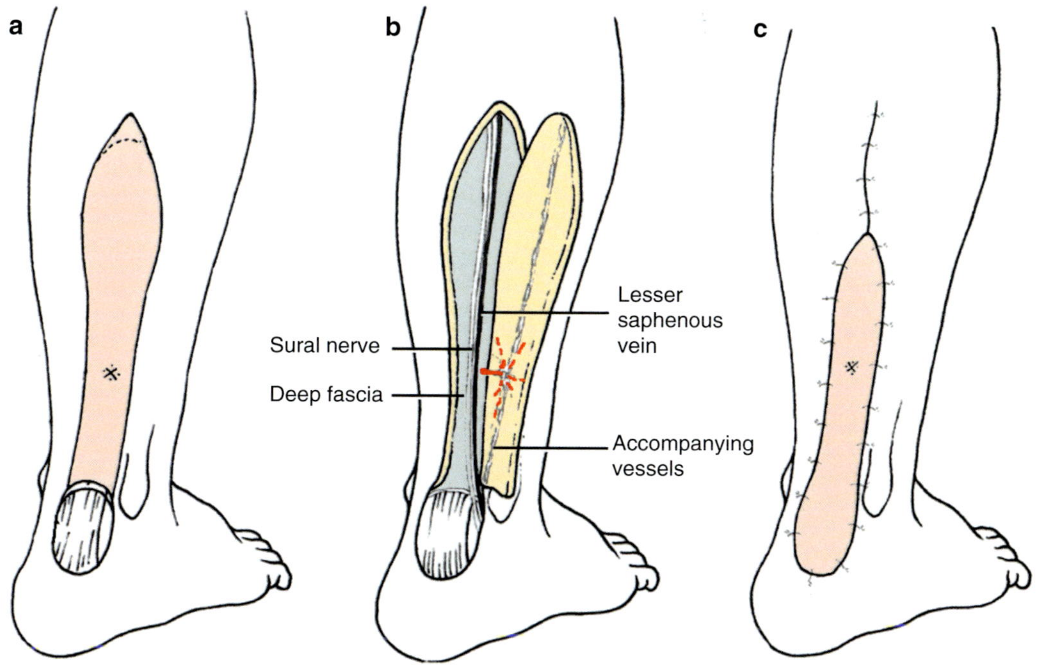

Fig. 4.3 Schematic drawing of perforator propeller flap (rotation)

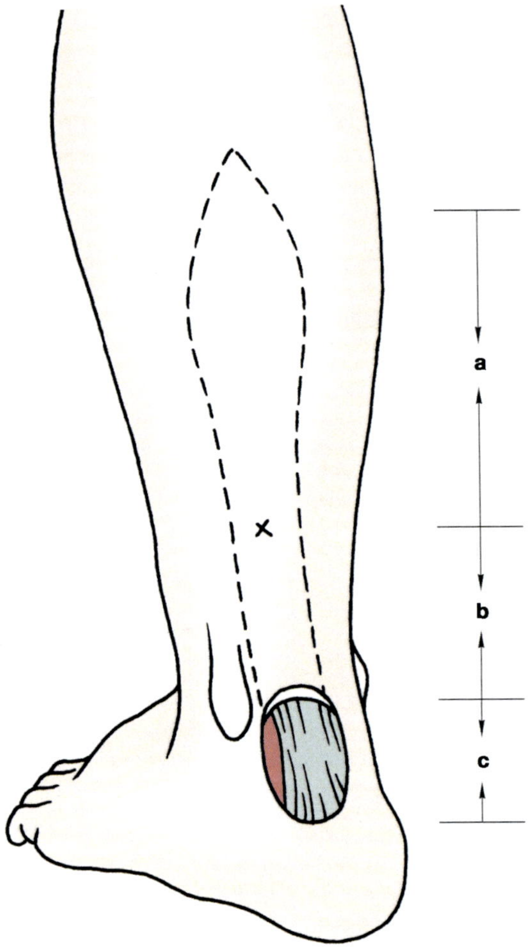

Fig. 4.4 Propeller flap design a > b+c

4.3.3 Rotation and Insetting of the Flap

Once the flap perfusion is satisfactory, it is ready to be rotated into the defect. The flap is carefully lifted from the wound bed, attached only by its pedicle, and rotated around this pedicle into the defect. The direction of rotation depends on the angle between the proximal long axis of the flap and the defect. This angle can be 90–180°. It is not necessary to rotate it beyond 180° because one can simply rotate the flap in the other direction. One may turn the flap into the defect clockwise and look closely at the pedicle, focusing on how comfortably the venae comitantes are positioned, looking in particular for any sign of kinking by any residual fascial strands which may need further division. And then turn the flap counterclockwise and do the same examination of the pedicle.

Once decided which rotational direction is the most comfortable, secure the flap into position with the first two skin sutures placed on either sides of the axis of the pedicle. These two sutures should be carefully positioned to ensure that the pedicle is not put under any traction tension either in a proximal or distal direction. If a suction drain is used, it is important to place it carefully under the flap and secured well away from pedicle. Thereafter, the rest of the flap inset and wound closure should be straightforward.

4.3.4 Donor-Site Closure

If the donor defect can be closed without excessive tension, that simplifies the final stages of the operation and produces the best esthetic result. One should however not be tempted to close the secondary defect of the wound so tightly, as such could risk the blood supply of the flap or causes swelling of the distal leg from a tourniquet effect. In that situation, a skin graft is preferable.

4.3.5 Which Is Better? Perforator Versus Perforator-Plus Pedicled

How to choose a pedicle in clinical practice? It depends on two factors: the finding of preoperative probing and the real intraoperative observation [5].

If a nice perforator is identified (caliber, length, perpendicular, good venous concomitants), we recommend microsurgical intraseptal dissection to skeletonize and complete free the perforator. It is a pure perforator-pedicled flap (Fig. 4.5).

If the perforator is not ideal, keep the septum and a quadrant adipofascial to protect the vessel and provide more venous drainage route. It is a perforator-plus-pedicled flap (Fig. 4.6).

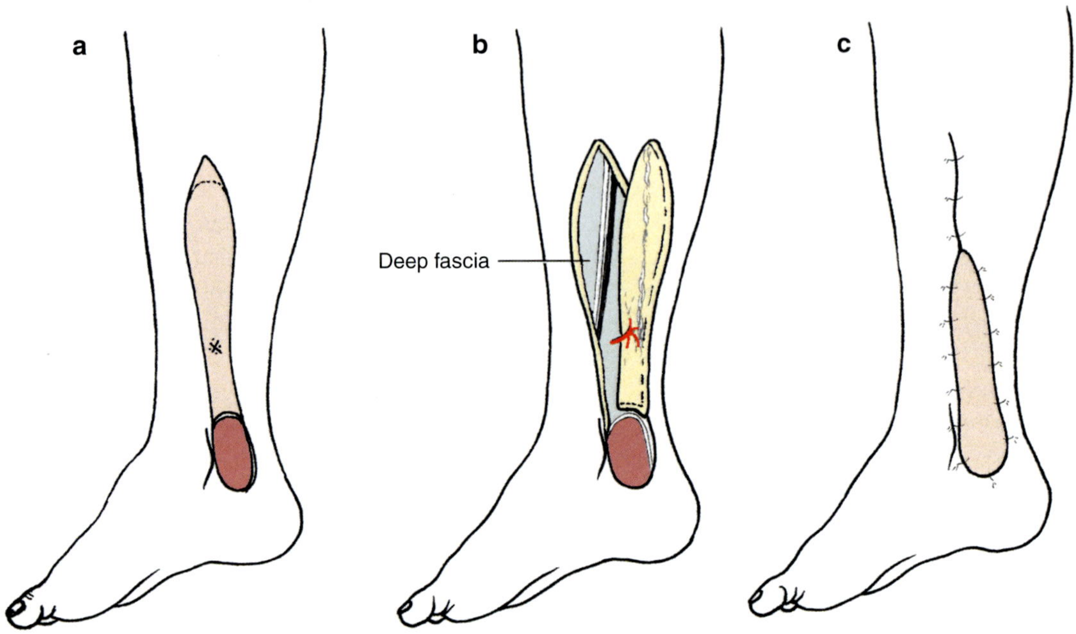

Fig. 4.5 True perforator-pedicled propeller flap. (**a**) Flap design, (**b**) flap elevation, (**c**) flap inset

Fig. 4.6 Perforator-plus-pedicled propeller flap. (**a**) Flap elevation, (**b**) flap inset

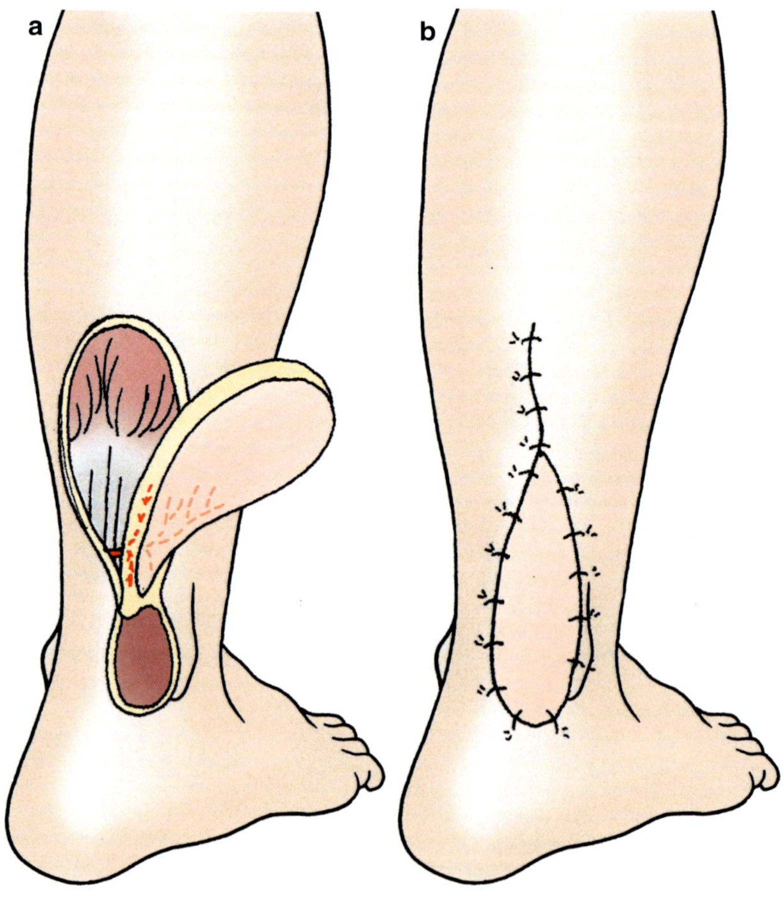

References

1. Hyakusoku H, Yamamoto Y, Fumiiri M. The propeller flap method. Br J Plast Surg. 1991;44(1):53–4.
2. Hyakusoku H, Ogawa R, Oki K, et al. The perforator pedicled propeller (PPP) flap method: report of two cases. J Nippon Med Sch. 2007;74(5):367–71.
3. Chang SM, Zhang F, Yu GR, Hou CL, Gu YD. Modified distally based peroneal artery perforator flap for reconstruction of foot and ankle. Microsurgery. 2004;24(6):430–6.
4. Chang SM, Tao YL, Zhang YQ. The distally perforator-pedicled propeller flap. Plast Reconstr Surg. 2011;128(5):575e–7.
5. Chang SM, Wang X, Huang YG, Zhu XZ, Tao YL, Zhang YQ. Distally based perforator propeller sural flap for foot and ankle reconstruction: a modified flap dissection technique. Ann Plast Surg. 2014;72(3):340–5.
6. Jakubietz RG, Jakubietz MG, Gruenert JG, et al. The 180-degree perforator-based propeller flap for soft tissue coverage of the distal, lower extremity: a new method to achieve reliable coverage of the distal lower extremity with a local, fasciocutaneous perforator flap. Ann Plast Surg. 2007;59(6):667–71.
7. Pignatti M, Pasqualini M, Governa M, et al. Propeller flaps for leg reconstruction. J Plast Reconstr Aesthet Surg. 2008;61(7):777–83.
8. Pignatti M, Ogawa R, Hallock GG, et al. The "Tokyo" consensus on propeller flaps. Plast Reconstr Surg. 2010;127(2):716–22.
9. Teo TC. The propeller flap concept. Clin Plast Surg. 2010;37:615–26.

5 Combined Perforator Flaps

There are five terms used by Hallock to name those complex flaps [1–3].

1. Compound flap. This consists of multiple and often diverse tissue components that are somehow joined together in a manner that will better allow their simultaneous transfer for a more efficient reconstruction. It can be further clarified into two major classes according to their intrinsic pattern of circulation.
2. *Composite* flap. This kind of compound flap has a *solitary* source of vascularization to all component parts, where this cannot be separated so all parts remain dependent on each other to insure viability. The traditional musculocutaneous or fasciocutaneous flaps are prime examples of this ubiquitous form of compound flap.
3. *Combined* flap. This kind of compound flap has *multiple* sources of vascularization, often discrete to each tissue component. The components of combined flaps can consist of any permutation of similar or non-similar tissues, which may be skin only, skin and muscle, muscle and bone, etc. The *combined* flap, in turn, can be further subdivided into two major subtypes that typically differ according to the physical relationship of their tissue components yet remain similar in that each of their parts retains an independent blood supply.
4. *Conjoined* flap, or Siamese flap. This kind of combined flap has multiple anatomical territories and is dependent to each other, due to some common physical junction, yet each retains an independent vascular supply.
5. *Chimeric* flap. This kind of combined flap consists of multiple parts, each with an independent vascular supply yet independent of any physical interconnection except where linked by a common vascular source.

C. Hou et al., *Surgical Atlas of Perforator Flaps: A Microsurgical Dissection Technique*,
DOI 10.1007/978-94-017-9834-1_5,

5.1 Conjoined Perforator Flap

This kind of flap has a large dimension and extends beyond a single perforasome. Each perforator independently nourishes its corresponding perforasome, yet each perforasome territory remains connected by a common border with the other. Clinically, there are two types: naturally indigenous and microsurgically fabricated (Fig. 5.1).

Indigenous conjoined perforator flaps can have perforators to their corresponding perforasomes that arise from a common source vessel or from independent branches that may even arise from different source vessels. A fabricated conjoined perforator flap will have the perforators within a given angiosome joined by an internal microanastomosis or, if from independent branches from the same or different angiosomes, joined together to form a congruent flap in a similar fashion connected to the terminus or a side branch of another.

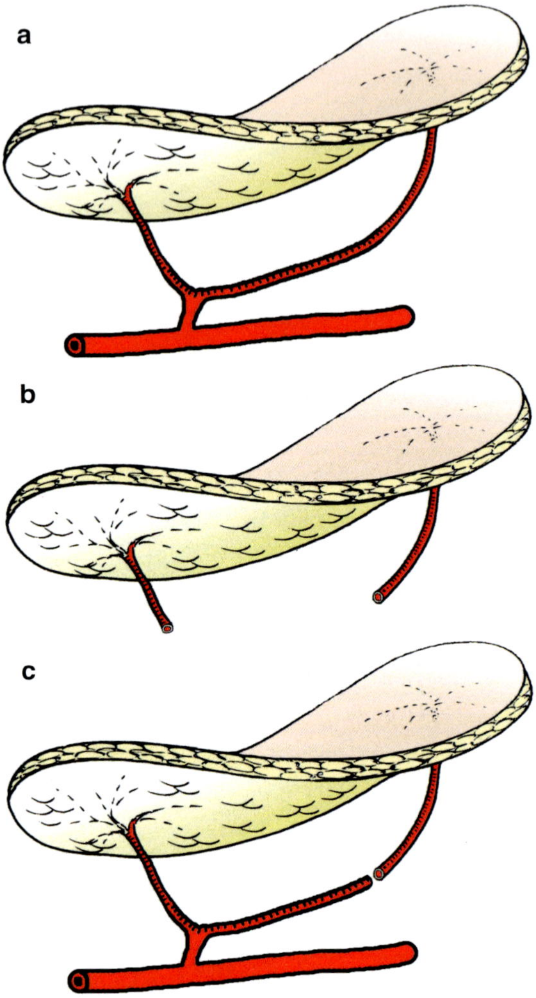

Fig. 5.1 Conjoined perforator flap. (**a**) Naturally indigenous, (**b**, **c**) microsurgically fabricated

5.2 Chimeric Perforator Flap

This kind of flap resembles a polyflap. If the tissue component of each flap is identical, it is called multi-paddled perforator flap (Fig. 5.2). If the tissue component is different, it is called chimeric perforator flap (Fig. 5.3).

If the boundaries between perforasomes of any naturally occurring conjoined perforator flap were split, with each territory remaining pedicled on its individual perforator, the resulting combined flap would become an *indigenous* type of perforator-based chimeric flap.

The independent perforasomes of indigenous chimeric perforator flaps are supplied by perforators that are ultimately connected by a common source vessel. Anatomical variations sometimes require an intraflap microanastomosis to fabricate an internal chimeric flap. In addition, otherwise discrete perforator flap source vessels can be connected to each other in a series to fabricate a sequential chimeric flap (Fig. 5.4).

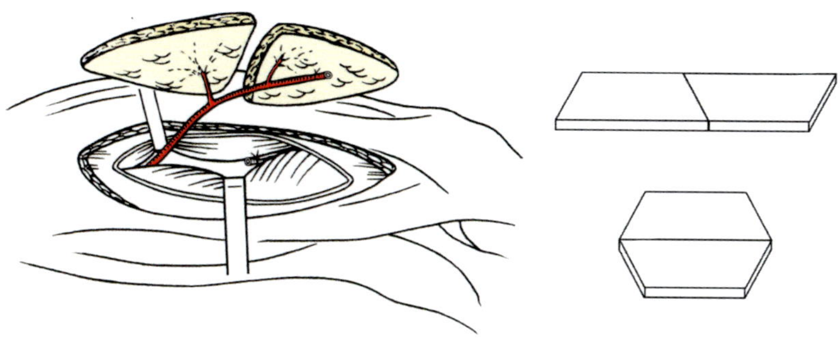

Fig. 5.2 Bi-paddled perforator flap

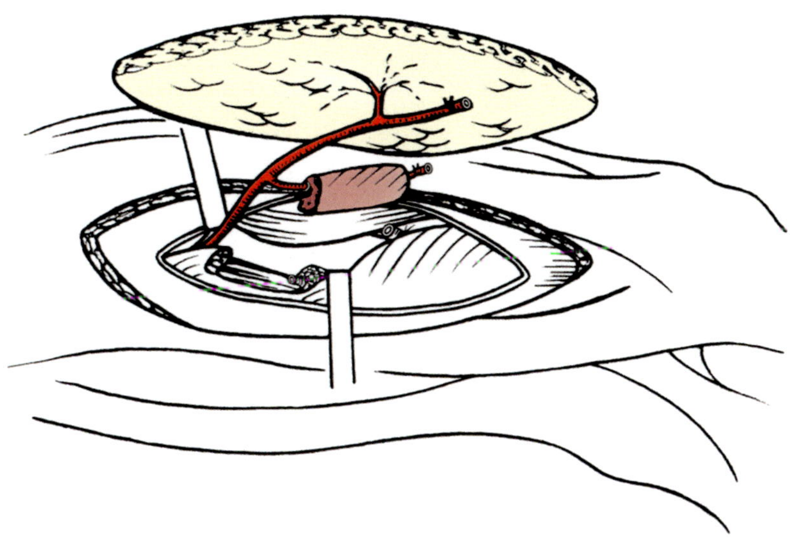

Fig. 5.3 Chimeric perforator flap

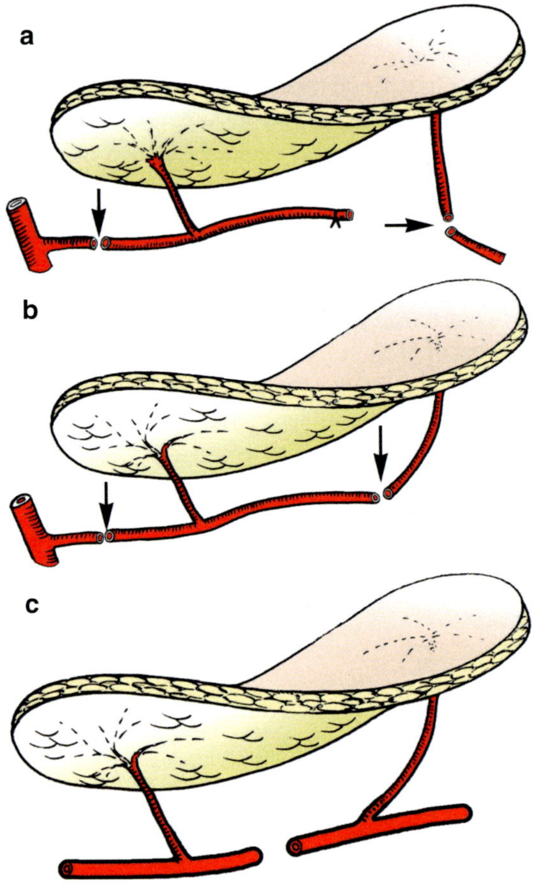

Fig. 5.4 Internal chimeric flap and sequential chimeric flap. (**a**) Internal chimeric flap, (**b**) fabricate internal chimeric flap, (**c**) sequential chimeric flap

References

1. Hallock GG. Simplified nomenclature for compound flaps. Plast Reconstr Surg. 2000;105:1465–70.
2. Hallock GG. Further clarification of the nomenclature for compound flaps. Plast Reconstr Surg. 2006;117:151e–60.
3. Hallock GG. The complete nomenclature for combined perforator flaps. Plast Reconstr Surg. 2011;127(4):1720–9.

6 Thinned Perforator Flaps

Bulky flaps cause aesthetically unacceptable outcomes and result in poor function in areas such as the feet, the hands, the face, and the neck. A thinned perforator flap suggests a uniformly thin adipose layer at the flap elevation. To simplify and avoid confusion in the nomenclature, the term thinned perforator flap is used to replace terms such as thin, super-thin, extremely thinned, and microdissected thin.

The thinned adipocutaneous perforator flap is based on the subdermal plexus, which is sensitive to excessive defatting and inappropriate flap design, especially when it is eccentric perforator based (Fig. 6.1).

C. Hou et al., *Surgical Atlas of Perforator Flaps: A Microsurgical Dissection Technique*,
DOI 10.1007/978-94-017-9834-1_6, © Springer Science+Business Media Dordrecht 2015

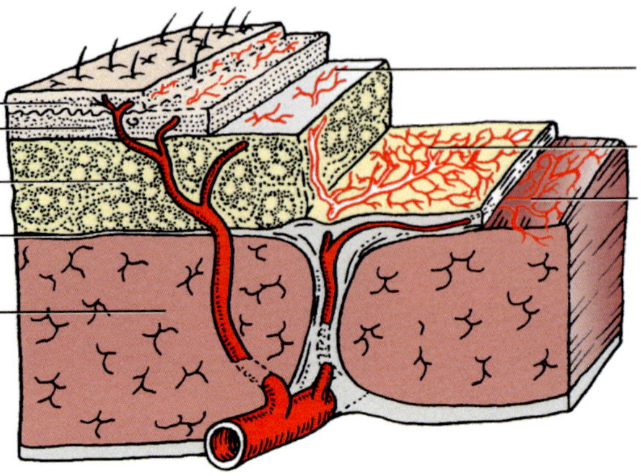

Fig. 6.1 The thinned perforator flap is nourished by the rich subdermal vascular plexus

6.1 Techniques of Defatting

Kimura [1] raised thin flaps by suprafascial dissection until the perforator was identified, and defatting was performed under a microscope to spare as much vascular branches as possible (Fig. 6.2).

Yang [2] introduced a modified microdissection technique, by harvesting the flap in a subfascial plane and performing a retrograde dissection of the perforator, later deferring the microdissection with a lower risk of traction injury.

The amount of deep fat lobules removed depends on the required thickness of the coverage defect. The adipofascial tissue is removed with tissue scissors, beginning from the periphery and stopping 1 cm from the location where the perforator enters the fat layer. To preserve subdermal plexus circulation, the superficial adipose layer, composed of the small and tight small fat lobules, should be preserved. The perforator entry is then dissected microscopically under tension. Those fat lobules intertwined with the perforator branches are then meticulously peeled off with microforceps. Direct dissection of perforator branches may injure tiny branches and is not recommended. Although some very tiny vessels to the fat lobules are visible in the microscopic field and may bleed when fat lobules are peeled off, the bleeding always stops spontaneously. After microdissection, the perforator branches are usually three to five in number in the adipose layer, which runs toward the subdermal plexus. Dissection is completed when the thickness of perforator entry is approximately the same as that in the periphery. During microdissection, irrigation with a heparin-containing solution should be continued to prevent desiccation.

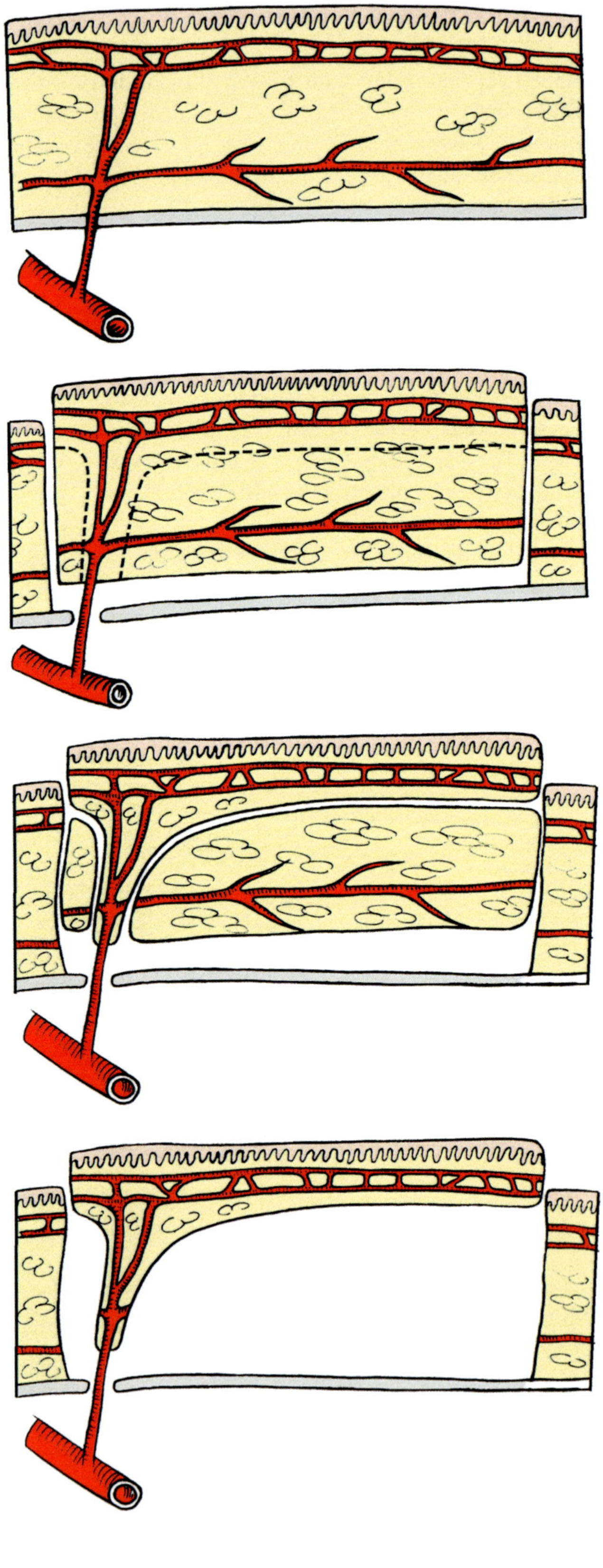

Fig. 6.2 Thinned adipocutaneous flap to the subdermal plexus. (**a**) Preservation of the deep fascia, deep compact adipose tissue, superficial fascia, and superficial loose adipose tissue. (**b**) Preservation of the loose superficial adipose tissue only. (**c**) Skeleton vascular pedicle according to the microdissection technique. (**d**) The final thinned flap

References

1. Kimura N, Satoh K. Consideration of a thin flap as an entity and clinical applications of the thin anterolateral thigh flap. Plast Reconstr Surg. 1996;97(5):985–92.
2. Yang WG, Chiang YC, Wei FC, Feng GM, Chen KT. Thin anterolateral thigh perforator flap using a modified perforator microdissection technique and its clinical application for foot resurfacing. Plast Reconstr Surg. 2006;117(3):1004–8.

Flow-Through Perforator Flaps

7

The concept of a flow-through flap, in which both the proximal and the distal ends of the vascular pedicle of a free flap are anastamosed to provide blood flow to distal tissues, was first described by Soutar et al. in 1983. Foucher et al. were the first to report the reconstruction of an extremity with a simultaneous vascular defect by utilizing a radial forearm flow-through flap in 1984.

The principle advantage of this flap is that it provides the opportunity for a single-stage composite reconstruction of both soft tissue and vascular defects, making it particularly useful in the reconstruction of ischemic extremities and defects from oncologic ablations and complicated trauma. Flow-through flaps can be classified from different point of inflow and outflow, orthograde and retrograde, and arterial and venous (Fig. 7.1) [1].

C. Hou et al., *Surgical Atlas of Perforator Flaps: A Microsurgical Dissection Technique*,
DOI 10.1007/978-94-017-9834-1_7, © Springer Science+Business Media Dordrecht 2015

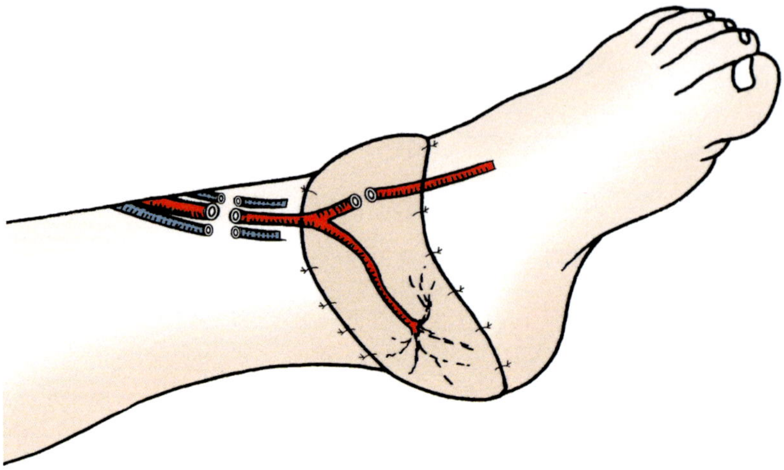

Fig. 7.1 Flow-through flap

Reference

1. Bullocks J, Naik B, Lee E, Hollier L Jr. Flow-through flaps: a review of current knowledge and a novel classification system. Microsurgery. 2006;26(6): 439–49.

Lateral Arm Perforator Flap

8

The lateral arm flap was first described by Song et al. in 1982 [1].

These indications have been well described by Katsaros et al. [2], Rivet et al. [3], and Scheker et al. [4] for reconstruction of the extremities and the head and neck.

8.1 Vascular Anatomy

The lateral upper arm flap is supplied by septocutaneous branches of the posterior radial collateral artery (PRCA), which develops from the profunda brachii artery. The perforators of the flap run within the lateral intermuscular septum, which separates the brachialis from the triceps muscle (Fig. 8.1).

In close proximity to the radial nerve, the vascular pedicle spirals around the humerus, and proximal to the lateral intermuscular septum, it divides into the small anterior and the stronger posterior radial collateral artery (PRCA). Whereas the small anterior radial collateral artery runs together with the radial nerve, the PRCA is the main nutrient artery of the flap, giving off the septocutaneous branches. After having traversed the septum at its base, the PRCA anastomoses with the interosseous recurrent artery, on which the flap can be perfused in a retrograde fashion.

The posterior cutaneous nerve of the arm (PCNA), which accompanies the PRCA, can be used to create sensate flaps [1, 5, 6].

Harvesting a cortical segment of the humerus is technically possible, but only to a size of 10×1 cm, leaving a muscle cuff on either side of the septum to include periosteal vessels of the PRCA [7].

C. Hou et al., *Surgical Atlas of Perforator Flaps: A Microsurgical Dissection Technique*,
DOI 10.1007/978-94-017-9834-1_8,

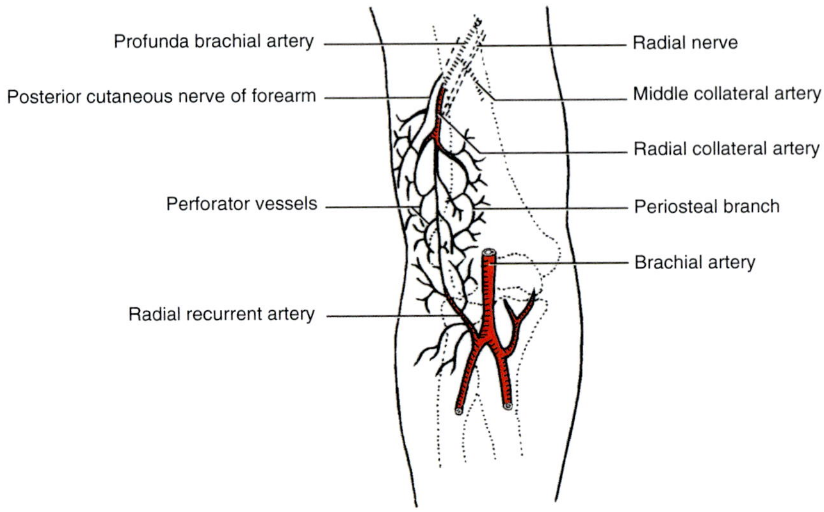

Fig. 8.1 Vascular anatomy of the lateral upper arm flap

8.2 Illustrative Case

A 33-year-old male underwent a traumatic severe crush injury of the left index finger. Emergency debridement was performed in another hospital. The patient refused to undergo toe pulp flap transplantation. So a free-arm flap was selected.

Flap Design

Draw a line from the insertion of the deltoid muscle to the lateral epicondyle of the humerus, corresponding to the lateral intermuscular septum (LIM), where the dominant pedicle and venae comitantes are found (Fig. 8.2). The perforator was identified preoperatively by using an 8 MHz handheld Doppler (Fig. 8.3).

Flap Elevation

Flap elevation began from the posterior side and moved toward the anterior side through the supracutaneous tissue plane. Once the perforator was identified, the lateral intermuscular septum was divided. The intermuscular septum and a tiny ellipse of deep fascia cuff were preserved around the radial collateral vessel and its skin perforator on the skin flap. The lateral cutaneous nerve of the arm was identified and contained in the flap. The entire flap was isolated (Fig. 8.4). Then, the pedicle of the flap was divided and ligated below the level at which the radial collateral artery was divided into anterior and posterior branches, at an average distance of 4 cm proximal to the lateral epicondyle (Fig. 8.5).

Flap Transfer

Finally, the flap was insetted into the defect (Fig. 8.6), followed by microsurgical anastomoses of posterior radial collateral artery and the venae comitantes.

All anastomoses were performed by using an end-to-end method (Fig. 8.7). The recipient arteries were the proper digital artery at the level of the proximal finger crease. Venous drainage occurred through the venae comitantes of posterior radial collateral artery. The recipient veins were the dorsal subcutaneous vein at the level of the proximal finger crease. Two vessels (an artery and a vein) were anastomosed. The lateral cutaneous nerve of the arm is sutured to the digital nerve as far distally as possible (Fig. 8.8).

The donor site was closed directly (Fig. 8.9). The donor site healed without any complications, and only a linear scar remained.

Follow-Up

The flap survived uneventfully (Fig. 8.10). No postoperative complication was detected.

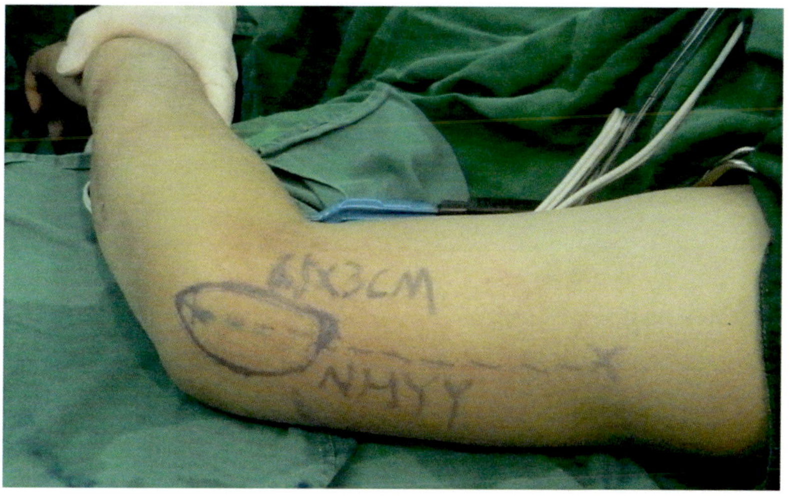

Fig. 8.2 Harvest a lateral arm perforator flap for finger coverage. (The case is offered by Professor Songlin Xie and Dr. Xiangwu Deng, Hand Surgical Centre, Nanhua Hospital, Nanhua University, Hengyang, China)

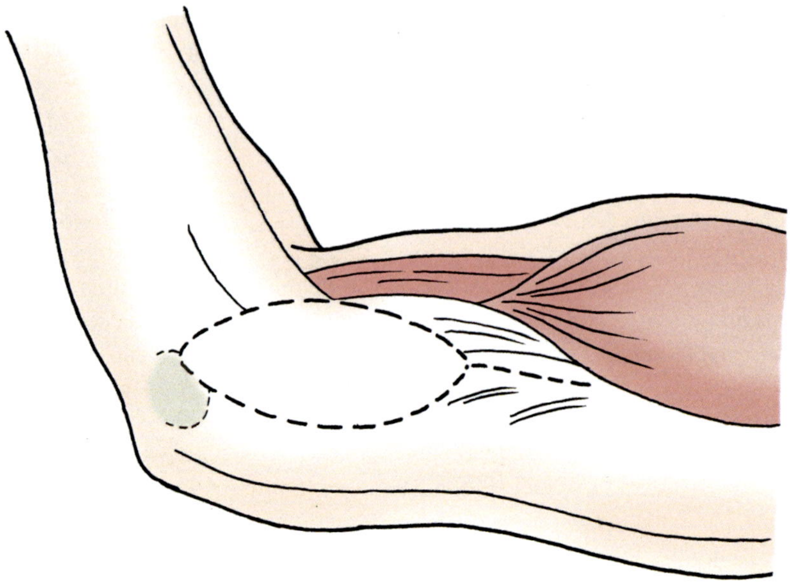

Fig. 8.3 Schematic drawing of the flap design

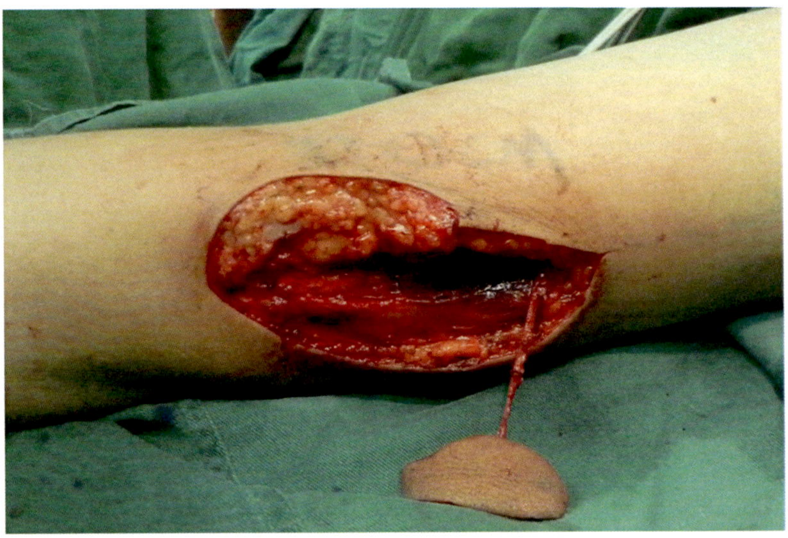

Fig. 8.4 The entire flap was isolated

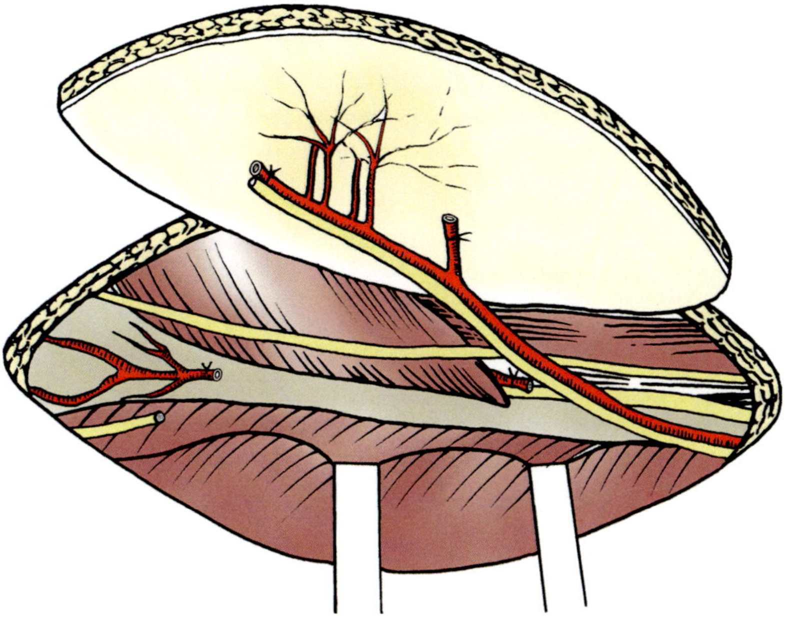

Fig. 8.5 Schematic drawing of the flap elevation

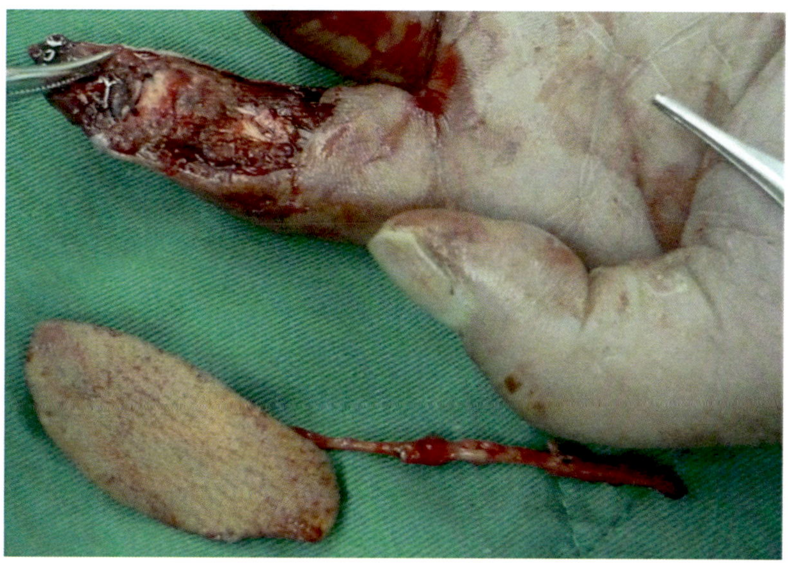

Fig. 8.6 The flap was transferred into the defect

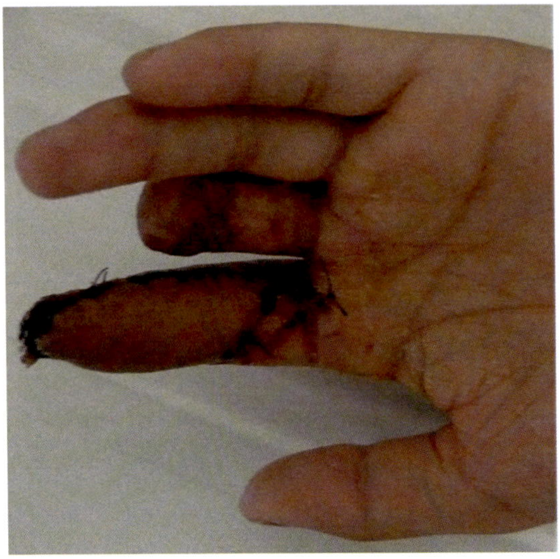

Fig. 8.7 Immediate postoperative view of the flap

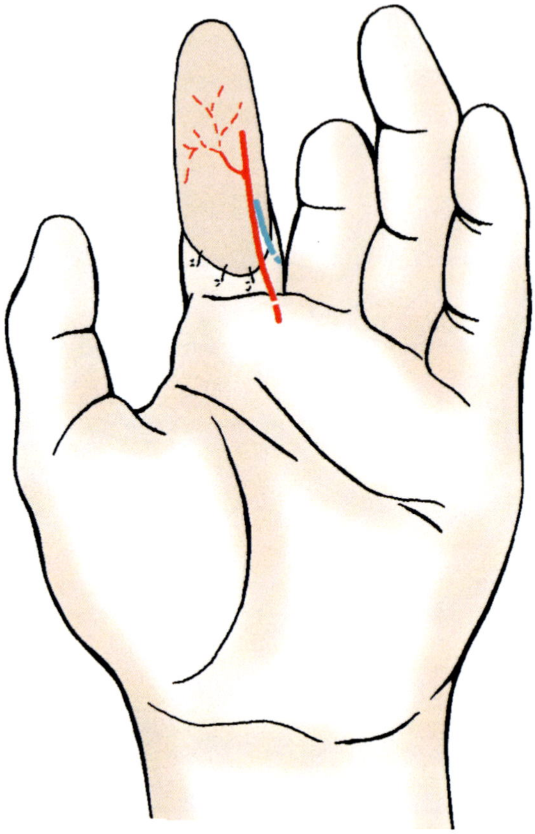

Fig. 8.8 Schematic drawing of flap blood supply rebuilding

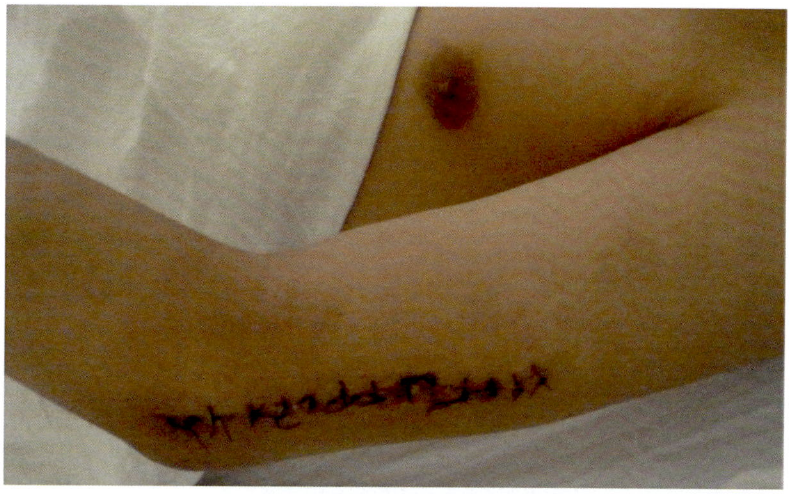

Fig. 8.9 The donor site was closed directly

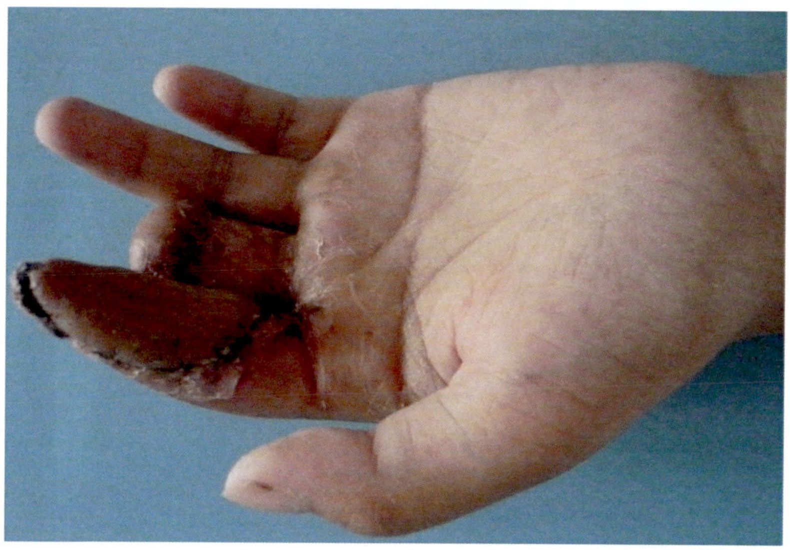

Fig. 8.10 Flap appearance in follow-up

Pearls

Donor site morbidity is limited to the ipsilateral upper extremity.

The lateral arm perforator flap does not sacrifice a major artery of the hand.

The flap can be raised with the patient in the supine position, which allows a more efficient two-team approach.

The osteofasciocutaneous variation of the lateral arm flap is ideally suited for reconstructing small bony defects such as those that occur with the metacarpals or metatarsals [8, 9].

The lateral upper arm flap has a reliable and constant anatomy, and because of the good color match and similar texture.

The possibility of creating sensate flaps is considered an advantage [5].

The lower lateral cutaneous nerve of the arm innervates this flap and can be sutured to a recipient sensory nerve, such as branches of the radial nerve, and provide protective sensation.

The combination of the skin paddle with a segment of the humerus bone or triceps muscle may contribute to a wider spectrum of indications for the flap [2, 7, 10, 11].

The high and reliable vascularity of the fascia allows for raising purely fascial flaps, which can be covered with split-thickness skin gra fts [1].

Pitfalls

The vascular pedicle might be missed if the septum is not incised directly at the humerus.

The vascular pedicle can easily be injured as it enters the flap at its cranial pole. Separate the pedicle from the radial nerve carefully, and place a loop around the vessels before the cranial pole of the flap is completely circumcised.

References

1. Song R, Song Y, Yu Y. The upper arm free flap. Clin Plast Surg. 1982;9(1):27–35.
2. Katsaros J, Schusterman M, Beppu M, Banis Jr JC, Acland RD. The lateral upper arm flap: anatomy and clinical applications. Ann Plast Surg. 1984;12(6):489–500.
3. Rivet D, Buffet M, Martin D, et al. The lateral arm flap: an anatomic study. J Reconstr Microsurg. 1987;3(2):121–32.
4. Scheker LR, Kleinert HE, Hanel DP. Lateral arm composite tissue transfer to ipsilateral hand defects. J Hand Surg. 1987;12(5 Pt 1):665–72.
5. Matloub HS, Larson DL, Kuhn JC, Yousif NJ, Sanger JR. Lateral arm free flap in oral cavity reconstruction: a functional evaluation. Head Neck. 1989;11(3):205–11.
6. Waterhouse N, Healy C. The versatility of the lateral arm flap. Br J Plast Surg. 1990;43(4):398–402.
7. Cormack GC, Lamberty BG. Fasciocutaneous vessels in the upper arm: application to the design of new fasciocutaneous flaps. Plast Reconstr Surg. 1984;74(2):244–50.
8. Haas F, Rappl T, Koch H, Pittler P, Scharnagl E. Free osteocutaneous lateral arm flap: anatomy and clinical applications. Microsurgery. 2003;23(2):87–95.
9. Hennerbichler A, Etzer C, Gruber S, Brenner E, Papp C, Gaber O. Lateral arm flap: analysis of its anatomy and modification using a vascularized fragment of the distal humerus. Clin Anat. 2003;16(3):204–14.
10. Song D, Xu J, Lv H, Liu J, Li J. Wraparound chimeric radial collateral artery perforator flap for reconstruction of thumb loss. J Reconstr Microsurg. 2015;31:95–101.
11. Liu J, Song D, Wu S, et al. (2014) Modified chimeric radial collateral artery perforator flap for repairing hand composite defects. J Reconstr Microsurg. 2015;31(3):171–8.

9 Medial Arm Perforator Flap

The reverse medial arm island flap is a local fasciocutaneous flap based on the recurrent ulnar artery [1].

The medial intermuscular septum is a very thick structure which feels like a tough cord. The brachial artery and median nerve run hugging the septum anteriorly, while the ulnar nerve does so posteriorly. These structures are identified and preserved while raising the flap [2–4].

9.1 Vascular Anatomy

The brachia artery is the continuation of the axillary artery beyond the teres major. The artery courses in the intermuscular septum between the biceps and the triceps (Fig. 9.1).

The profunda artery is a musculocutaneous artery that is usually the first branch off the brachial. It arises 2–3 cm beyond the teres major and passes posteriorly between the humerus and the triceps to accompany the radial nerve. The branches from the profunda brachii supply the triceps and then perforate into the skin. Small cutaneous branches perforate the muscular fascia at 2 to 3 cm intervals, to supply the skin of the posterior two-thirds of the arm.

The superior ulnar collateral artery is an axial cutaneous vessel that arises 4–6 cm beyond the pectoralis major and courses distally through the subcutaneous tissue to enter the medial arm skin 6–12 cm beyond the pectoralis. The arterial diameter is from 0.8 to 1.5 mm. In 60 % of dissections this artery originates from the profunda artery, and in 20 % it originates directly from the brachial artery. In the other 20 % there is a double system with a direct cutaneous vessel exiting from both the brachial artery and the profunda artery. In this latter situation the vessel size is inadequate for free flap transfer but can be used for local or distant pedicle flaps.

The biceps musculocutaneous artery arises 6–8 cm distal to the pectoral muscle. After penetrating the biceps muscle, two or three major perforating vessels vascularize the anterior arm skin. The size of these vessels is variable.

The inferior ulnar collateral artery is an axial cutaneous artery that arises 5–10 cm from the elbow and may form collaterals either around the elbow or with the superior ulnar collateral artery. In 6 out of 16 dissections, a 0.4–0.6 mm direct cutaneous artery supplied the skin of the distal third of the arm.

C. Hou et al., *Surgical Atlas of Perforator Flaps: A Microsurgical Dissection Technique*,
DOI 10.1007/978-94-017-9834-1_9, © Springer Science+Business Media Dordrecht 2015

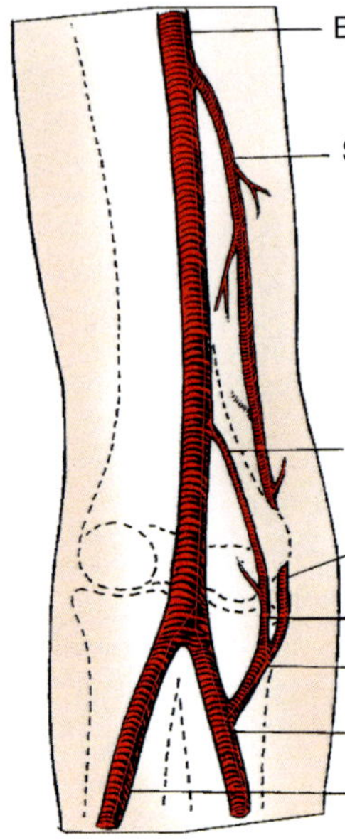

Fig. 9.1 Vascular anatomy of the medial arm flap

9.2 Illustrative Case

A 43-year-old man suffered from severe crush injury of his right upper extremity from machine accident. The forearm was unreplantable. A distally based flap was designed to cover the amputated stump (Fig. 9.2).

Flap Design

The flap pivot is located above the medial epicondyle; the largest perforator is located approx. 10 cm proximally of the medial epicondyle in the palpable medial intermuscular septum (Fig. 9.3).

Preoperative flap planning includes both identification of the superior ulnar collateral artery, using the Doppler flow meter, and marking of the large subcutaneous veins. The flap is centered along the axis of the superior ulnar brachial cutaneous collateral artery, as determined by Doppler, and includes at least one large superficial vein (Fig. 9.4).

Flap Elevation

The anterior incision is first made and the deep fascia divided 0.5 cm. away from the skin. The flap is now raised at the subfascial level until the medial intermuscular septum is reached. The brachial artery and the median nerve are identified as they run hugging the septum and gently dissected off it. The posterior incision is now made and the fascia over the triceps. The flap is now elevated at the subfascial level until the ulnar nerve is identified running close to the medial intermuscular septum. The nerve is separated from the septum and the two incisions, anterior and posterior, are joined in an arc.

The skin boundaries are incised down through and including the areolar plane overlying the muscular fascia. The deep plane of elevation includes the areolar fascia to protect the superior brachial collateral artery. Dissection on the muscular fascia can be rapid until the point of penetration of the vessel into the skin, beginning distally at the flap tip, as determined by the Doppler study (about 6–10 cm from the anterior axillary fold). Care is taken to avoid the intermuscular septum that contains the ulnar rand median nerves and the brachia/ artery. Protection is facilitated by marking the brachial artery course between the biceps and triceps. Proximal to the point where the superior ulnar collateral artery penetrates the skin, the dissection requires more care, so as not to transect this direct cutaneous artery as it exits the intermuscular septum (Fig. 9.5). The dissection is terminated as soon as enough elevation has been completed to allow transfer to the recipient site (Fig. 9.6).

Flap Transfer

The flap was rotated 180° to cover the extremity stump (Fig. 9.7). The donor site was closed directly.

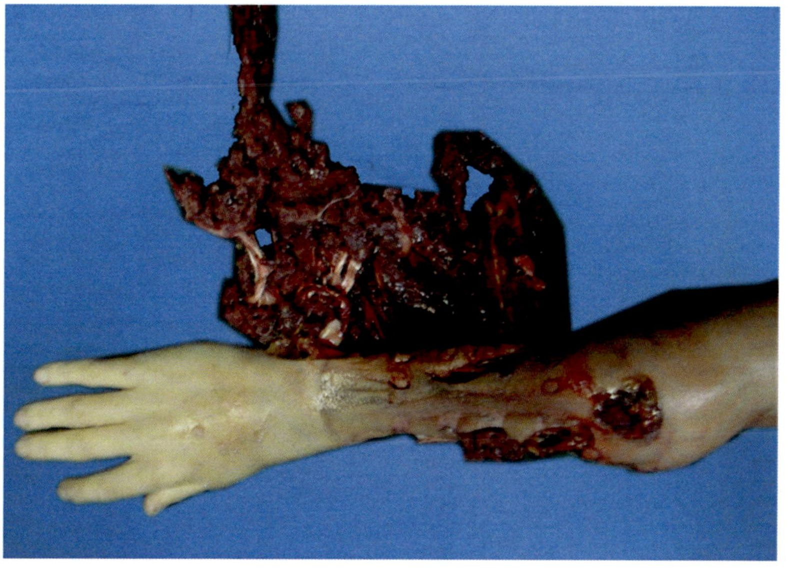

Fig. 9.2 Preoperative view

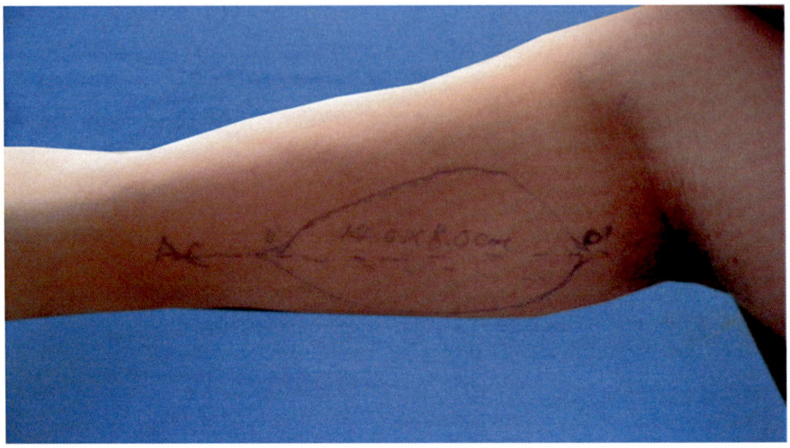

Fig. 9.3 Flap design

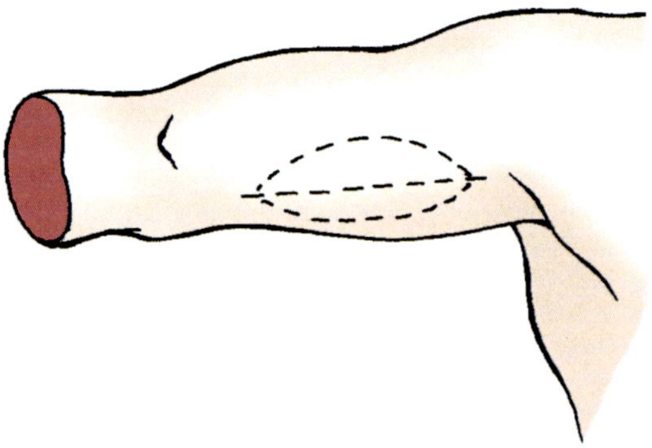

Fig. 9.4 Schematic drawing of flap design

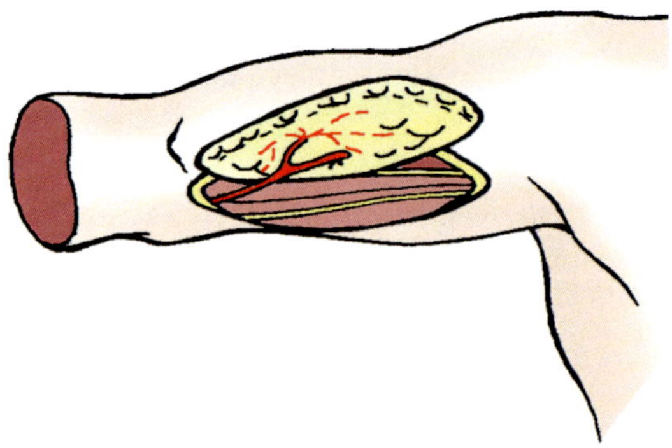

Fig. 9.6 Schematic drawing of the flap raising

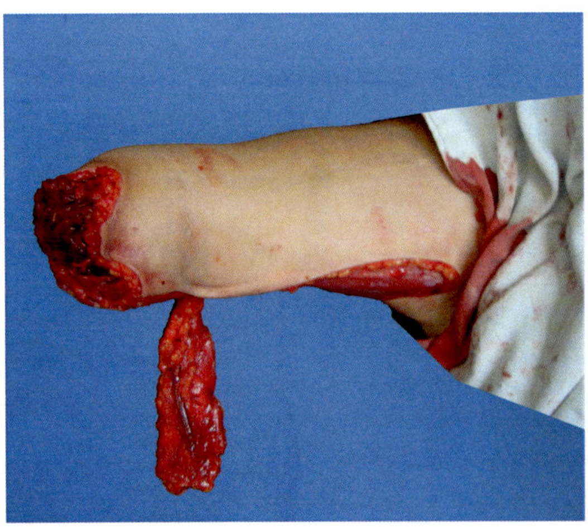

Fig. 9.5 Flap elevation

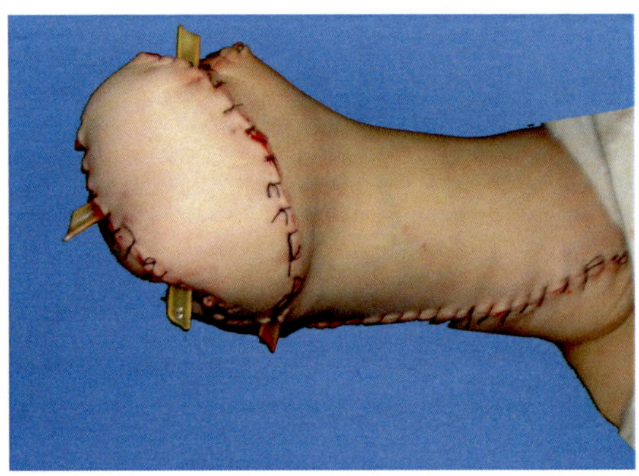

Fig. 9.7 Flap transfer

Pearls

Medial arm skin is very thin, elastic, and hairless.

The donor site is well hidden and no functional problem.

Medial arm septocutaneous perforator flaps can be used for release of axillary and elbow-crease contractures and can be deepithelialized for contour improvement of the anterior axillary wall and for subclavicular depression after mastectomy.

Pitfalls

It can be used as a direct, distant, or free flap, depending on the recipient site. By including the medial brachial cutaneous nerve, the free flap can also provide protective sensation.

References

1. Daniel RK, Terzis J, Schwarz G. Neurovascular free flaps. A preliminary report. Plast Reconstr Surg. 1975;56(1):13–20.
2. Kaplan EN, Pearl RM. An arterial medial arm flap–vascular anatomy and clinical applications. Ann Plast Surg. 1980;4(3):205–15.
3. Karamursel S, Bagdatli D, Demir Z, Tuccar E, Celebioglu S. Use of medial arm skin as a free flap. Plast Reconstr Surg. 2005;115(7):2025–31.
4. Newsom HT. Medical arm free flap. Plast Reconstr Surg. 1981;67(1):63–6.

10 Radial Artery Perforator Flap

The reverse-flow radial forearm (Chinese) island flap is based on a distal vascular pedicle consisting of the radial artery and its venae comitantes. The advantages of using this pedicled flap for hand reconstruction are numerous. However, two major disadvantages of the donor site restrict the flap's clinical applications. First, the sacrifice of a major artery may possibly jeopardize hand viability. Second, a displeasing scar deformity may occur if split-skin grafts are used for closure. Surgeons have made efforts to overcome these drawbacks. The distally based radial forearm perforator flap—a new flap based on the tiny perforators around the radial styloid process and the longitudinal chain-linked vascular plexuses—was invented.

The radial artery perforator (RAP) flap with preservation of the radial artery was firstly reported by Zhang [1] for hand reconstruction. Chang [2] performed an anatomic study in 1990 to show that the pivot point of the pedicle was located 1.5 cm proximal to the radial styloid process.

C. Hou et al., *Surgical Atlas of Perforator Flaps: A Microsurgical Dissection Technique*,
DOI 10.1007/978-94-017-9834-1_10,

10.1 Vascular Anatomy

Along its course down the forearm, the radial artery gives off approximately 12 perforators to the skin along the fascial septum [3].

These perforators arise between the brachioradialis and pronator teres muscles in the proximal third of the forearm and between the brachioradialis and flexor carpi radialis muscles in the distal two-thirds. Distally, one or two of these perforators may be between the tendons of the flexor carpi radialis and flexor digitorum superficialis muscles. These forearm perforators within the fascial plexus are oriented predominantly along the longitudinal axis in the forearm and transversely in the carpal [4, 5]. The distal radial artery issued about ten small branches (0.3–0.8 mm in diameter) extending from 1.5 cm above the radial styloid process to the bifurcation of the radial artery. These perforators pass through the septum, fan out on both surfaces of the deep fascia, and form a rich, chain-linked longitudinal plexus of the integument along the course of the main artery, the septum, the fiber of the deep fascia, and the superficial vein. The venous system of the deep fascia drains blood to the profunda venae comitantes directly through the concomitant perforating veins. The distal pivot point of the pedicle was located 1.0–1.5 cm proximal to the radial styloid process (Fig. 10.1).

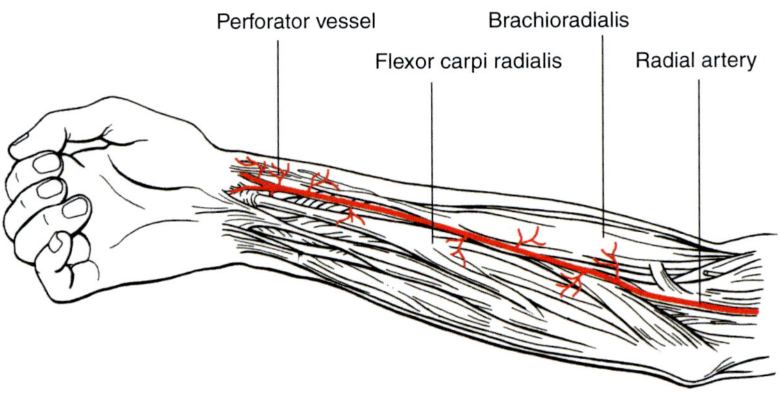

Fig. 10.1 Vascular anatomy of the radial artery

10.2 Illustrative Case

Case 1: Proximal Perforator-Based Flap

A 29-year-old man was involved in an industrial accident that resulted in an injury to the distal third of his dorsal forearm, with tendon and skin loss (Fig. 10.2).

Flap Design (Fig. 10.3)

A distally based radial forearm fasciocutaneous flap, from the radial aspect of the middle-third forearm and nourished by a perforator from the middle radial artery, was designed to cover the defect. The flap size was 12 by 8 cm (Fig. 10.4).

The flap was elevated and visualized the perforator vessels (Figs. 10.5 and 10.6).

Flap Transfer

The flap was transferred to cover the defect. The donor-site wound was resurfaced with a split-thickness graft (Fig. 10.7).

Follow-Up

The flap survived smoothly (Fig. 10.8).

Case 2: Radial Styloid Perforator-Based Flap

An injury to this 27-year-old man's hand resulted in soft tissue defects on the dorsum of the thumb (Fig. 10.9).

Flap Design (Fig. 10.10)

A 10×3 cm radial forearm perforator flap without radial artery was designed in the distal two-thirds of the forearm. The distal perforator pedicle was located 2 cm proximal to the radial styloid process (Fig. 10.11).

Flap Elevation

After identifying the distal perforator, a 3 cm wide adipofascial was kept around the tiny vessel to prevent it from stretching. It is a perforator-plus flap (Fig. 10.12).

Flap Transfer and Insetting

The flap was rotated 180° to cover the defect. The donor site was closed with skin grafts (Fig. 10.13).

Follow-Up

The flap survived smoothly (Fig. 10.14).

Case 3: Snuff Box Perforator-Based Flap

This 32-year-old man presented with injuries to the extensor tendon and soft tissue of the dorsal hand of the 2nd metacarpal head. Bone was exposed. The injuries were caused by an accident involving farming machinery.

Flap Design

The distally based radial forearm fasciocutaneous flap is vascularized by the perforators of the distal radial artery. The skin flap is along the axis of the radial artery; the pivot point of its adipofascial pedicle (usually 3 cm in width) is located at the snuff box (a snuff box perforator). The flap size was 8 by 3 cm (Figs. 10.15 and 10.16).

Flap Elevation

After identifying the distal perforator, a 3 cm wide adipofascial was kept around the tiny vessel to prevent it from stretching (Fig. 10.17).

Flap Transfer and Insetting

The flap was rotated 180° to cover the defect. The donor-site wound was covered with a split-thickness graft (Fig. 10.18).

Follow-Up

The flap healed well, without complications (Fig. 10.19).

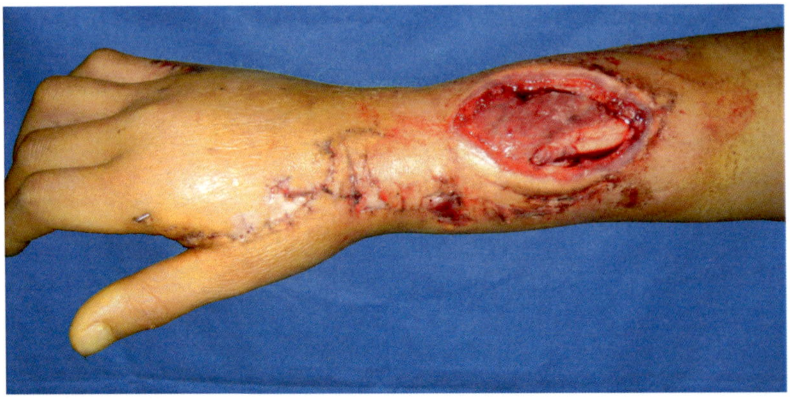

Fig. 10.2 Preoperative view

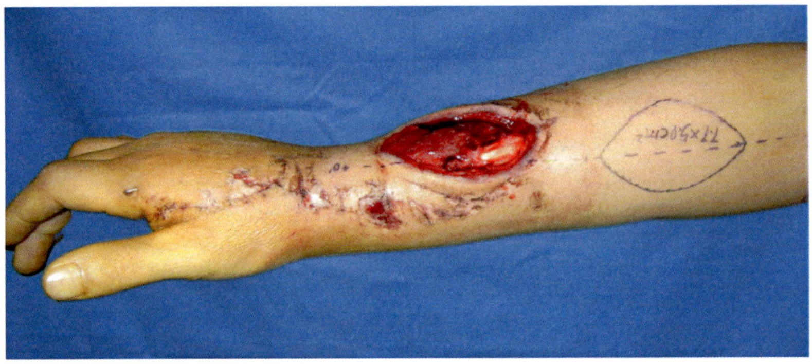

Fig. 10.3 Flap design

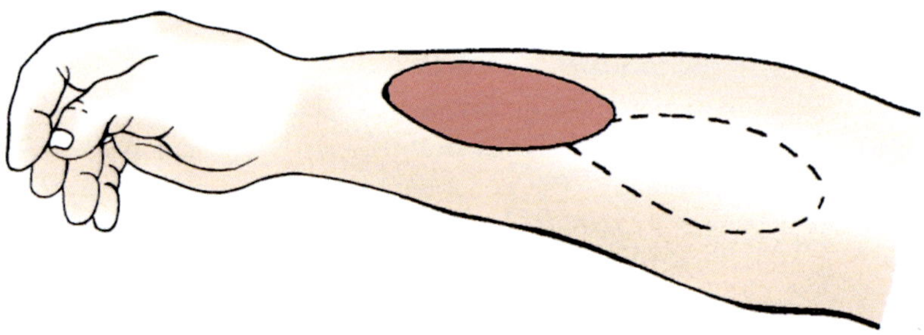

Fig. 10.4 Schematic drawing of the flap design

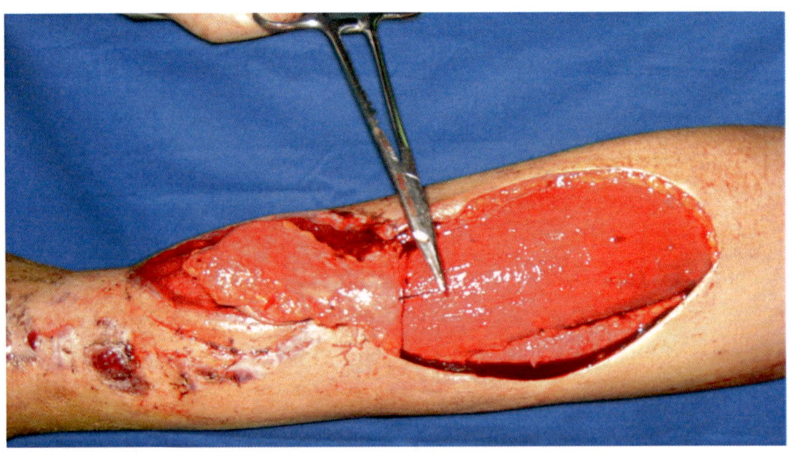

Fig. 10.5 Flap elevation

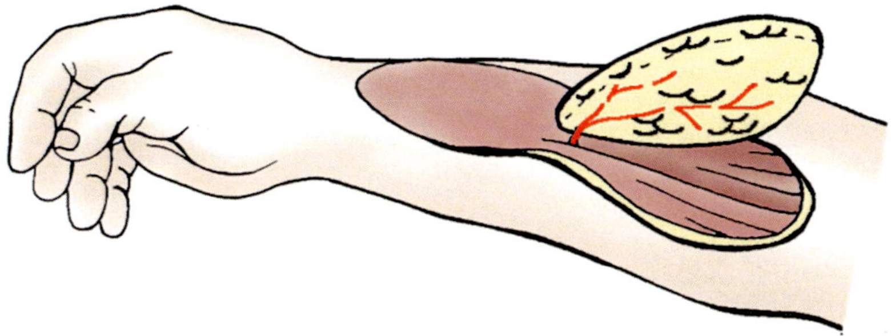

Fig. 10.6 Schematic drawing of the flap elevation

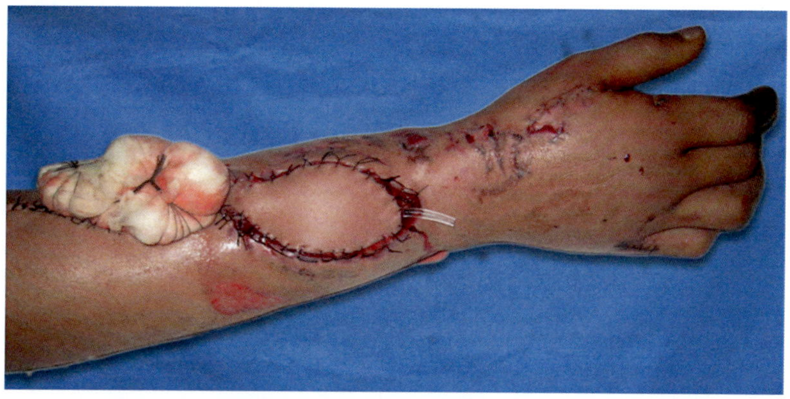

Fig. 10.7 Flap transfer

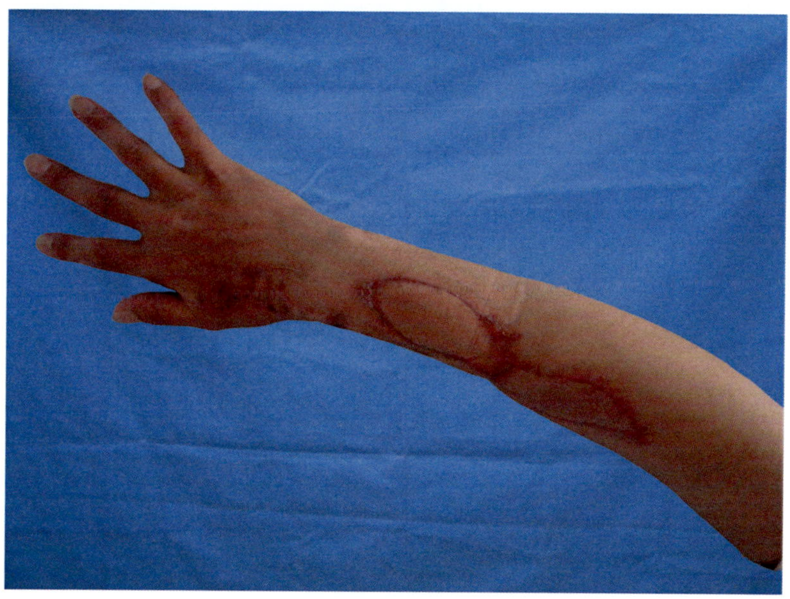

Fig. 10.8 Follow-up

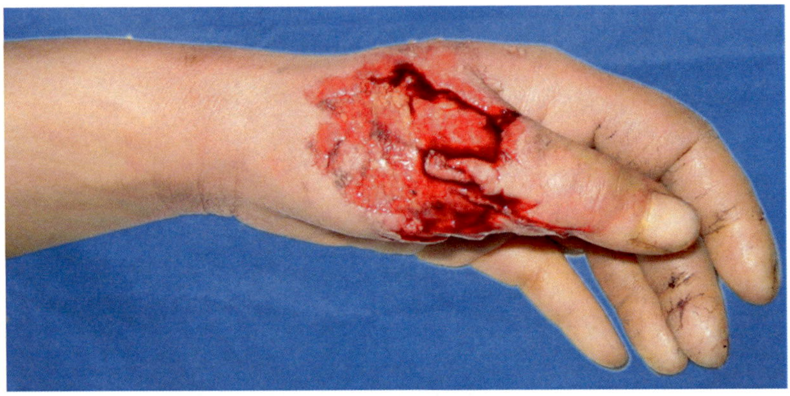

Fig. 10.9 Preoperative view

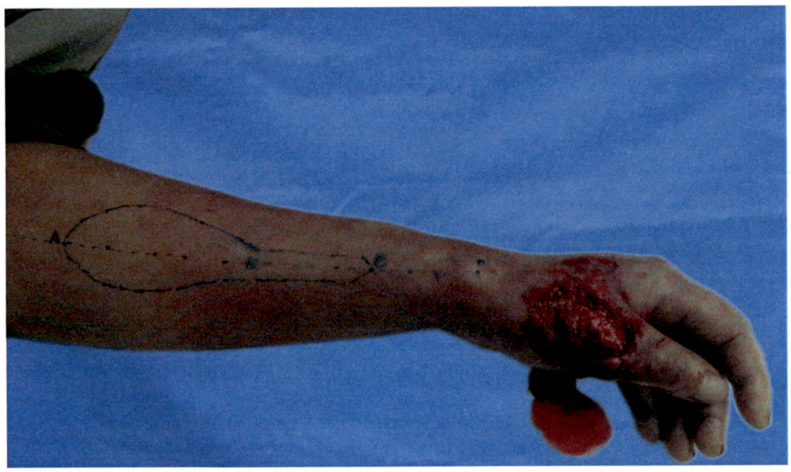

Fig. 10.10 Flap design

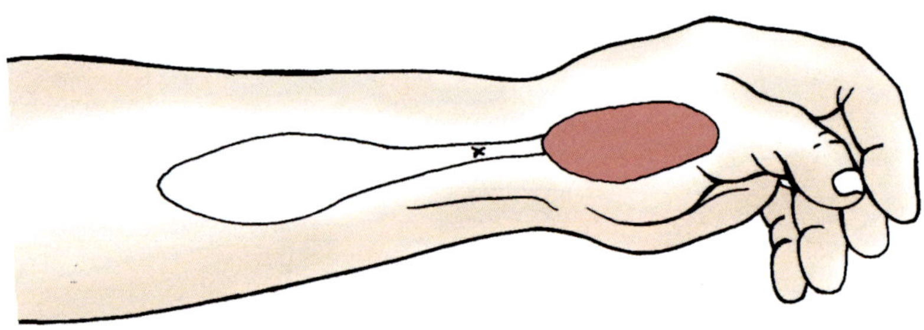

Fig. 10.11 Schematic drawing of flap design

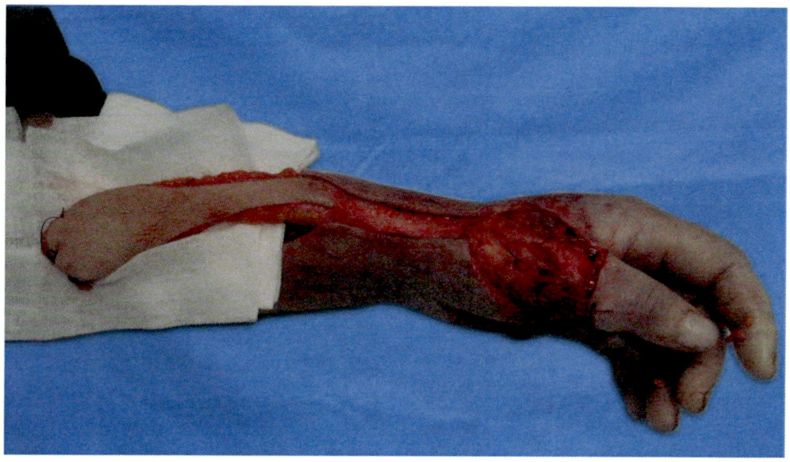

Fig. 10.12 Flap elevation

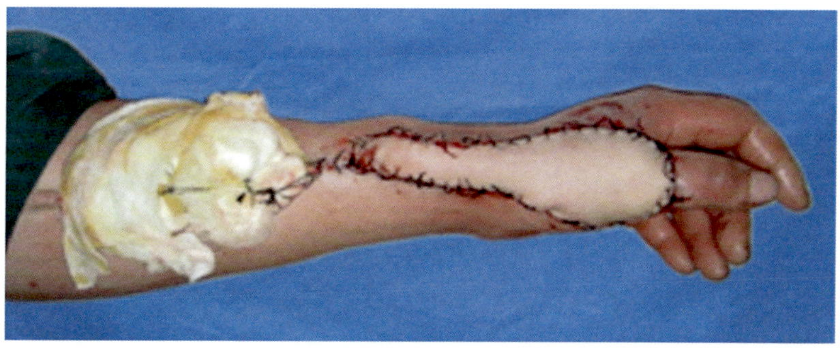

Fig. 10.13 Flap transfer and insetting

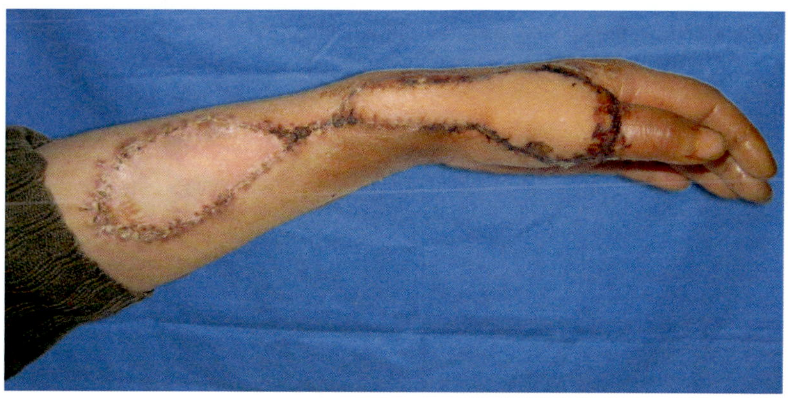

Fig. 10.14 Follow-up

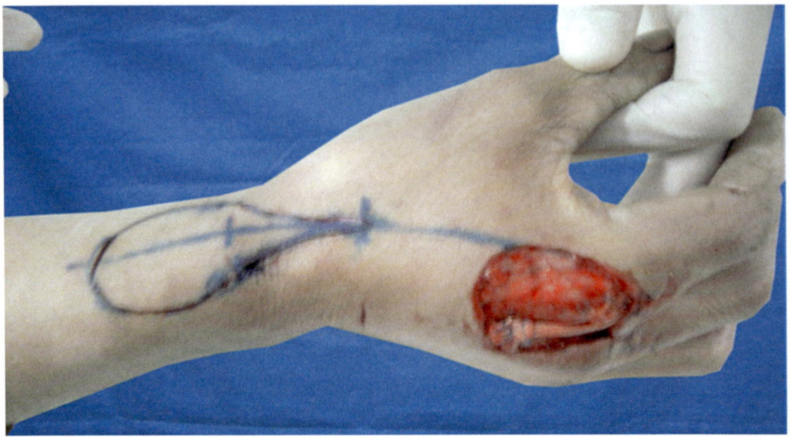

Fig. 10.15 Preoperative view and flap design

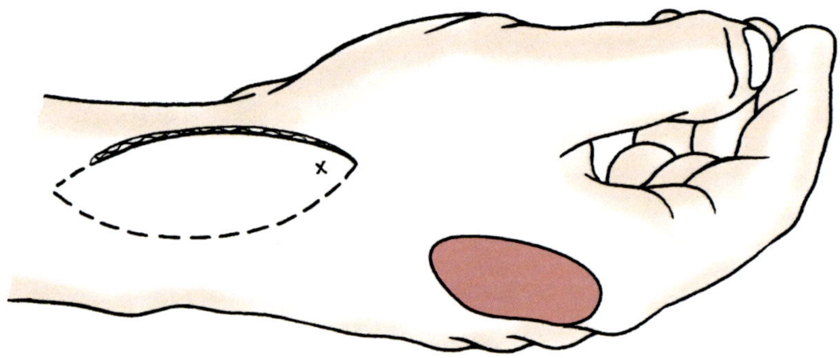

Fig. 10.16 Schematic drawing of flap design

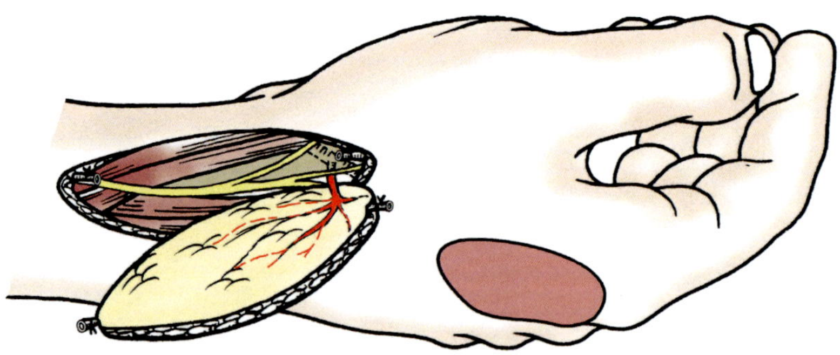

Fig. 10.17 Flap elevation

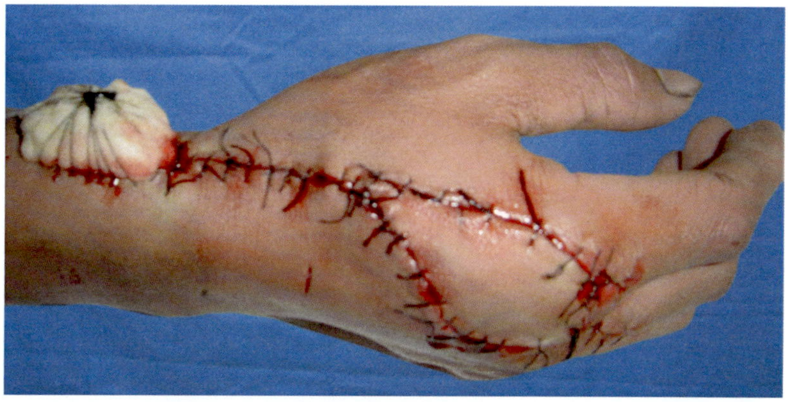

Fig. 10.18 Flap transfer and insetting

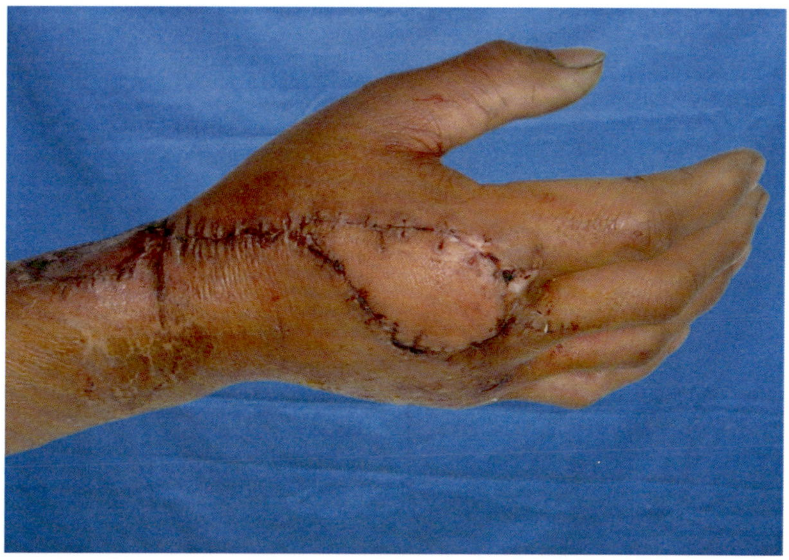

Fig. 10.19 Follow-up

Pearls

The flap is easy to raise and transfer and does not require microsurgical techniques [6].

This flap not only preserves the radial artery but also provides a more acceptable donor site [7].

The flap has constant and reliable blood supply with preservation of the main radial artery [3, 8–10].

This flap could potentially be used as an innervated flap, with the inclusion of the lateral cutaneous nerve of the forearm [11–13].

Composite flaps from the radial forearm including other tissues, such as the periosteum, tendon, and nerve, can also be harvested [14–21].

Pitfalls

The RAP flap is generally based on a single perforator, either proximally or distally [12, 22].

The proximally based radial forearm fasciocutaneous flap, based on the inferior cubital artery, may be used as a local perforator flap or as a microvascular free flap [23–27].

References

1. Zhang YT. The use of reversed forearm pedicled fascio-cutaneous flap in the treatment of hand trauma and deformity (report of 10 cases). Zhonghua Zheng Xing Shao Shang Wai Ke Za Zhi. 1988;4(1):41–2.
2. Chang SM. The distally based radial forearm fascia flap. Plast Reconstr Surg. 1990;85(1):150–1.
3. Yang D, Morris SF, Tang M, Geddes CR. Reversed forearm island flap supplied by the septocutaneous perforator of the radial artery: anatomical basis and clinical applications. Plast Reconstr Surg. 2003;112(4):1012–6.
4. Kanellakos GW, Yang D, Morris SF. Cutaneous vasculature of the forearm. Ann Plast Surg. 2003;50(4):387–92.
5. Inoue Y, Taylor GI. The angiosomes of the forearm: anatomic study and clinical implications. Plast Reconstr Surg. 1996;98(2):195–210.
6. Fang QG, Shi S, Zhang X, Li ZN, Liu FY, Sun CF. Upper extremity morbidity after radial forearm flap harvest: a prospective study. J Int Med Res. 2014;42(1):231–5.
7. Xu LQ, Fan QY, Zhang BL, Zhang H, Zhang CP, Hu GH. Establishment of hemodynamic model of human radial forearm free flap. Shanghai Kou Qiang Yi Xue. 2011;20(2):136–40.
8. Weinzweig N, Chen L, Chen ZW. The distally based radial forearm fasciosubcutaneous flap with preservation of the radial artery: an anatomic and clinical approach. Plast Reconstr Surg. 1994;94(5):675–84.
9. Koshima I, Moriguchi T, Etoh H, Tsuda K, Tanaka H. The radial artery perforator-based adipofascial flap for dorsal hand coverage. Ann Plast Surg. 1995;35(5):474–9.
10. Jeng SF, Wei FC. The distally based forearm island flap in hand reconstruction. Plast Reconstr Surg. 1998;102(2):400–6.
11. Liu WW, Li H, Guo ZM, et al. Reconstruction of soft-tissue defects of the head and neck: radial forearm flap or anterolateral thigh flap? Eur Arch Otorhinolaryngol. 2011;268(12):1809–12.
12. Song C, Wong M, Wong CH, Ong YS. Modifications of the radial forearm flap phalloplasty for female-to-male gender reassignment. J Reconstr Microsurg. 2011;27(2):115–20.
13. Song M, Chen SW, Zhang Q, et al. External monitoring of buried radial forearm free flaps in hypopharyngeal reconstruction. Acta Otolaryngol. 2011;131(2):204–9.
14. Medalie DA. Perforator-based forearm and hand adipofascial flaps for the coverage of difficult dorsal hand wounds. Ann Plast Surg. 2002;48(5):477–83.
15. Safak T, Akyurek M. Free transfer of the radial forearm flap with preservation of the radial artery. Ann Plast Surg. 2000;45(1):97–9.
16. Koshima I, Tsutsui T, Nanba Y, Takahashi Y, Akisada K. Free radial forearm osteocutaneous perforator flap for reconstruction of total nasal defects. J Reconstr Microsurg. 2002;18(7):585–8; discussion 589–90.
17. Zhou W, He M, Liao Y, Yao Z. Reconstructing a complex central facial defect with a multiple-folding radial forearm flap. J Oral Maxillofac Surg. 2014;72(4):836.e1–4.
18. Lee JT, Chen PR, Cheng LF, et al. A comparison between proximal lateral leg flap and radial forearm flap for intraoral reconstruction. Ann Plast Surg. 2013;71 Suppl 1:S43–7.
19. Li YY, Sun JE, Li G, Liang M. Reconstructing a full-thickness cheek defect of electrical burn with a folding radial forearm flap. J Oral Maxillofac Surg. 2013;71(10):1811.e1–3.
20. Cheng YS, Li WL, Xu L, Xu ZF, Liu FY, Sun CF. Assessment of quality of life of oral cancer patients after reconstruction with radial forearm free flaps. Zhonghua Kou Qiang Yi Xue Za Zhi. 2013;48(3):161–4.

21. Li W, Xu Z, Liu F, Huang S, Dai W, Sun C. Vascularized free forearm flap versus free anterolateral thigh perforator flaps for reconstruction in patients with head and neck cancer: assessment of quality of life. Head Neck. 2013;35(12):1808–13.
22. Tan NC, Lin PY, Kuo PJ, et al. An objective comparison regarding rate of fistula and stricture among anterolateral thigh, radial forearm, and jejunal free tissue transfers in circumferential pharyngo-esophageal reconstruction. Microsurgery. 2014;17(6):356–9.
23. Fang QG, Li ZN, Zhang X, Liu FY, Xu ZF, Sun CF. Clinical reliability of radial forearm free flap in repair of buccal defects. World J Surg Oncol. 2013;11:26.
24. Lee JC, Hsu WT, Yang CC, Chang SH. A fabricated forearm free flap with accompanying phonation tube for simultaneous reconstruction of a pharyngolaryngeal circumferential defect and voice loss: new surgical modification with functional phonation outcome. Laryngoscope. 2013;123(2):344–9.
25. Liu Y, Zhao YF, Huang JT, et al. Analysis of 13 cases of venous compromise in 178 radial forearm free flaps for intraoral reconstruction. Int J Oral Maxillofac Surg. 2012;41(4):448–52.
26. Chen Y, Zhang K, Li J, Xu J, Liao S, Xu T. Early effectiveness of combining radial forearm free flap and adjacent tissue flap in reconstruction of palatomaxillary defects. Zhongguo Xiu Fu Chong Jian Wai Ke Za Zhi. 2011;25(9):1051–4.
27. Chang SM, Hou CL, Zhang F, et al. Distally based radial forearm flap with preservation of the radial artery: anatomic, experimental and clinical studies. Microsurgery. 2003;23(4):328–37.

11 Ulnar Artery Perforator Flap

Lovie et al. [1] originally described the ulnar artery forearm flap as a free flap in 1984.

The true ulnar artery perforator (UAP) flap includes skin from the ulnar forearm or hand based on an ulnar artery perforator, with preservation of the ulnar artery. In the distal third of the forearm, an island flap based on a single dorsal perforator of the ulnar artery has been used. Becker and Gilbert [2] described a flap from the ulnar border of the distal dorsal forearm based on the dorsal branch of the ulnar artery.

11.1 Vascular Anatomy

The ulnar artery territory passes around the ulnar border of the forearm, extending onto the dorsal surface to the subcutaneous border of the ulna. Most of the perforators longitudinally anastomose with each other along the course of the main artery. These perforators form a deep fascial plexus and are arranged longitudinally along the main arterial axis.

In the distal third of the forearm, the ulnar artery gives off its dorsal branch 2–7 cm proximal to the pisiform bone. The distally based dorsal UAP flap is outlined on the dorsal ulnar aspect of the distal forearm. The potential area of the flap is 6 by 16 cm, with the length extending from the distal third of the forearm to the distal third of the dorsal surface of the hand [3]. The flap can be used for reconstructing the palm, dorsum, or ulnar border of the hand [4–8].

The dorsal branch of the ulnar artery runs obliquely from the palmar to the dorsal surface, passing deep to the flexor carpi ulnaris muscle and superficial to the ulnar nerve. It then gives off a fasciocutaneous branch that divides into an ascending branch and a descending branch (Fig. 11.1).

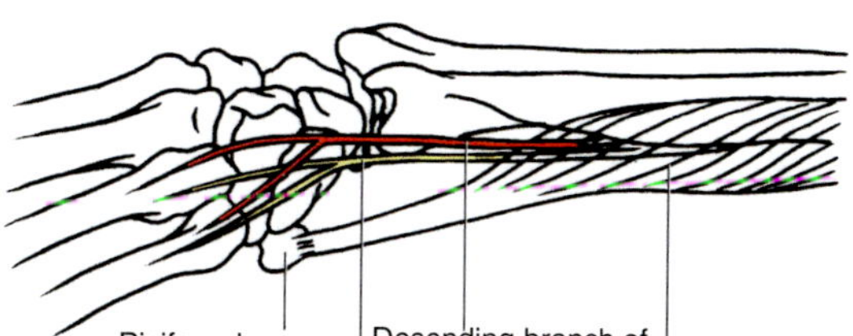

Fig. 11.1 Vascular anatomy of ulnar artery and nerve

C. Hou et al., *Surgical Atlas of Perforator Flaps: A Microsurgical Dissection Technique*,
DOI 10.1007/978-94-017-9834-1_11, © Springer Science+Business Media Dordrecht 2015

11.2 Illustrative Case

This 35-year-old man's right hand was crushed in an industrial ice machine and was managed elsewhere with dressings for several weeks (Fig. 11.2).

Flap Design

The flap measured 10×4.5 cm. The incision site was outlined on the ulnar side of the wrist and forearm overlying the tendon of flexor carpi ulnaris muscle (Fig. 11.3). The pisiform was identified and the pedicle was located emerging between 2 and 5 cm from it (Fig. 11.4).

Flap Elevation

The dorsal branch of the ulnar artery is dissected in the wrist, and it is ligated close to its origin. The fasciocutaneous flap is then dissected in a proximal to distal direction (Fig. 11.5). The deep fascia should be included in the flap, and the distally based pedicle is elevated with the subcutaneous tissue to preserve the anastomosis (Fig. 11.6).

Flap was attached with the donor site only by the perforator (Fig. 11.7).

Flap Insetting

The flap was rotated 180° to reconstruct defects on the dorsum of the hand without disrupting the ulnar artery (Fig. 11.8).

Follow-Up

The flap survived smoothly. The ultimate outcome was satisfactory, with a functional range of motion (Fig. 11.9).

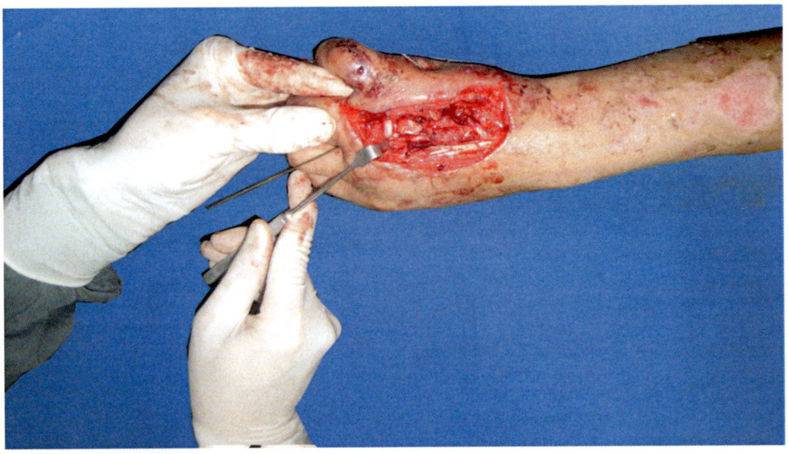

Fig. 11.2 Preoperative view

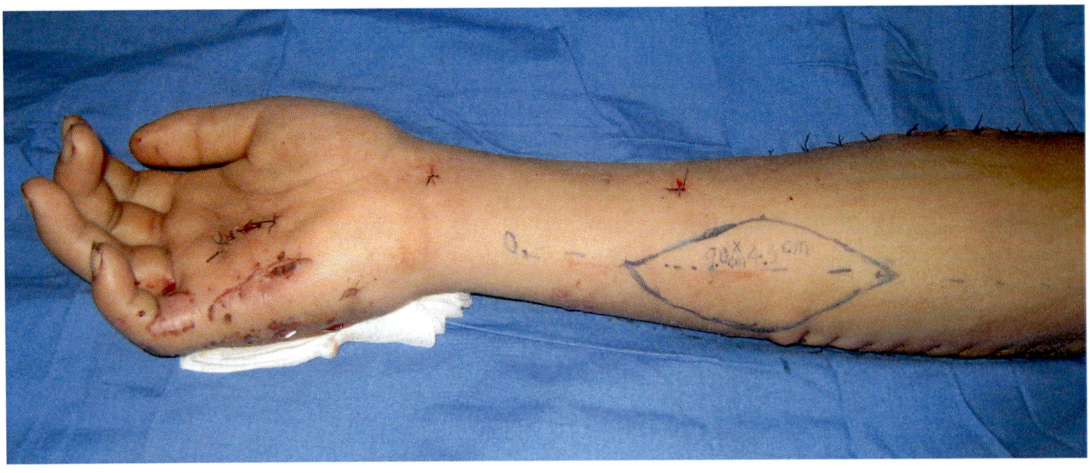

Fig. 11.3 Flap design

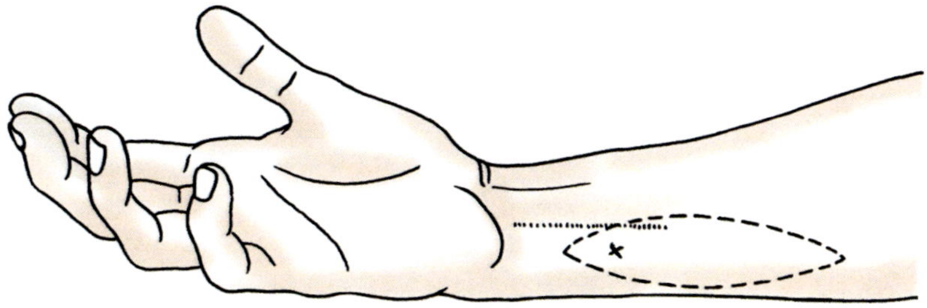

Fig. 11.4 Schematic drawing of flap design

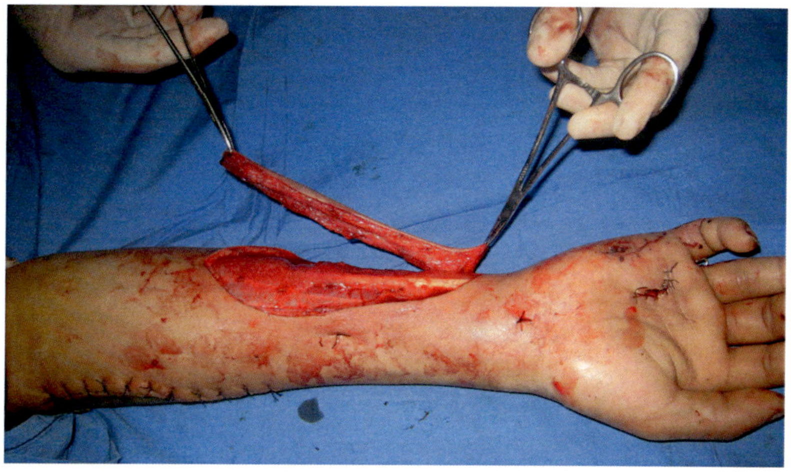

Fig. 11.5 Flap elevation

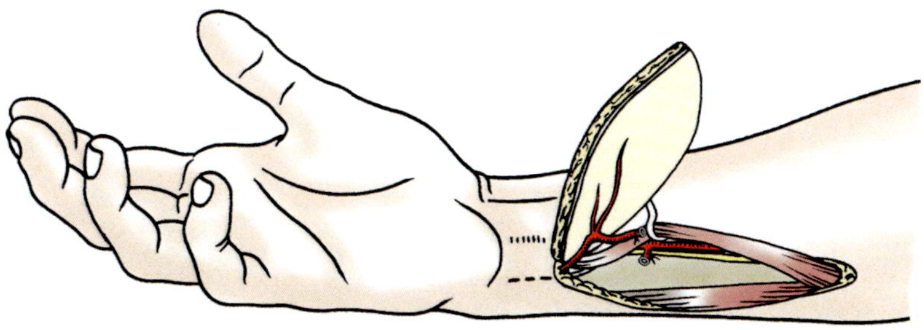

Fig. 11.6 Schematic drawing of the flap elevation

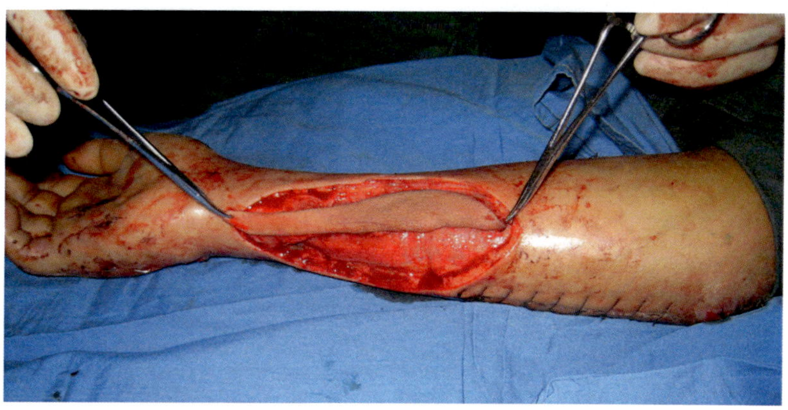

Fig. 11.7 Flap rotation

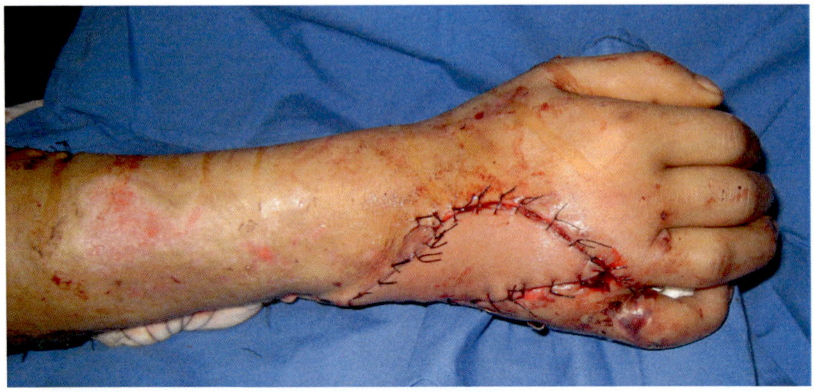

Fig. 11.8 Flap insetting

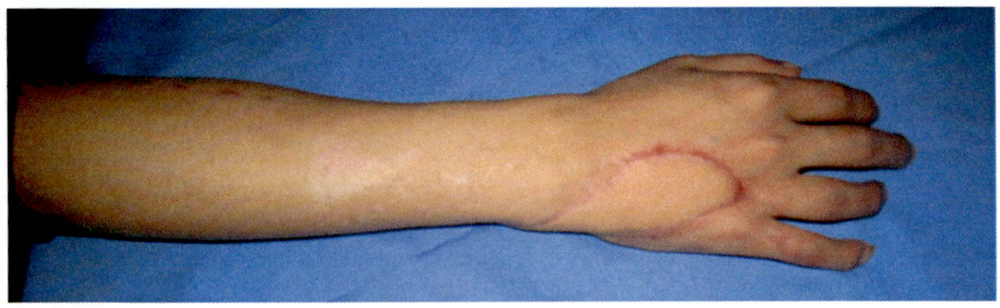

Fig. 11.9 Follow-up

Pearls

The UAP flap offers several advantages such as ease of donor site closure, cosmetic acceptability, and hairlessness [9, 10].

Pitfalls

Important considerations in harvesting a UAP flap are the variable location and size of the artery's perforators. A Doppler examination alone is often inadequate for predicting the location and size of the perforators.

To obtain a greater arc of rotation, the flap can be designed more proximally, based on the ascending branch of the dorsal branch of the ulnar artery in a subcutaneous pedicle flap [11].

If insufficient vascularity is noted in the elevated dorso-ulnar flap after the tourniquet is released, the elevated flap should be converted from a reverse pedicled flap to a free flap.

References

1. Lovie MJ, Duncan GM, Glasson DW. The ulnar artery forearm free flap. Br J Plast Surg. 1984;37(4):486–92.
2. Becker C, Gilbert A. The ulnar flap. Handchir Mikrochir Plast Chir. 1988;20(4):180–3.
3. Bertelli JA, Pagliei A. The neurocutaneous flap based on the dorsal branches of the ulnar artery and nerve: a new flap for extensive reconstruction of the hand. Plast Reconstr Surg. 1998;101(6):1537–43.
4. Karacalar A, Ozcan M. Preliminary report: the distally pedicled dorsoulnar forearm flap for hand reconstruction. Br J Plast Surg. 1999;52(6):453–7.
5. Ignatiadis IA, Mavrogenis AF, Avram AM, et al. Treatment of complex hand trauma using the distal ulnar and radial artery perforator-based flaps. Injury. 2008;39 Suppl 3:S116–24.
6. Liu DX, Wang H, Li XD, Du SX. Three kinds of forearm flaps for hand skin defects: experience of 65 cases. Arch Orthop Trauma Surg. 2011;131(5):675–80.
7. Sauerbier M, Unglaub F. Perforator flaps in the upper extremity. Clin Plast Surg. 2010;37(4):667–76, vii.
8. Page R, Chang J. Reconstruction of hand soft-tissue defects: alternatives to the radial forearm fasciocutaneous flap. J Hand Surg. 2006;31(5):847–56.
9. Koshima I, Iino T, Fukuda H, Soeda S. The free ulnar forearm flap. Ann Plast Surg. 1987;18(1):24–9.
10. Christie DR, Duncan GM, Glasson DW. The ulnar artery free flap: the first 7 years. Plast Reconstr Surg. 1994;93(3):547–51.
11. Karacalar A, Ozcan M. Use of a subcutaneous pedicle ulnar flap to cover skin defects around the wrist. J Hand Surg. 1998;23(3):551–5.

Posterior Interosseous Artery Perforator Flap

12

The posterior interosseous artery flap was firstly introduced by Zancolli and Angrigiani [1] and Penteado et al. [2].

The reverse pedicle posterior interosseous artery perforator (PIOAP) flap is an extremely useful tool for hand coverage.

12.1 Vascular Anatomy

The posterior interosseous artery courses distally in the septum between the extensor digiti minimi and extensor carpi ulnaris muscles and gives off interstitial arteries (usually 3–8 septocutaneous perforators) that run perpendicular to the skin on the dorso-ulnar aspect of the forearm [3].

The distally based posterior interosseous artery pedicle flap is based on a direct communication to the dorsal branches of the anterior interosseous artery, which is 2.5 cm above the wrist level. This direct anastomosis is a very consistent finding that was confirmed in 97.1–100 % of cadaveric limbs [2, 4–8]. The distal-most perforator, located 2–3 cm above the ulnar styloid process, is usually selected as the pivot point for distal PIA perforator-based flap for hand reconstruction (Fig. 12.1).

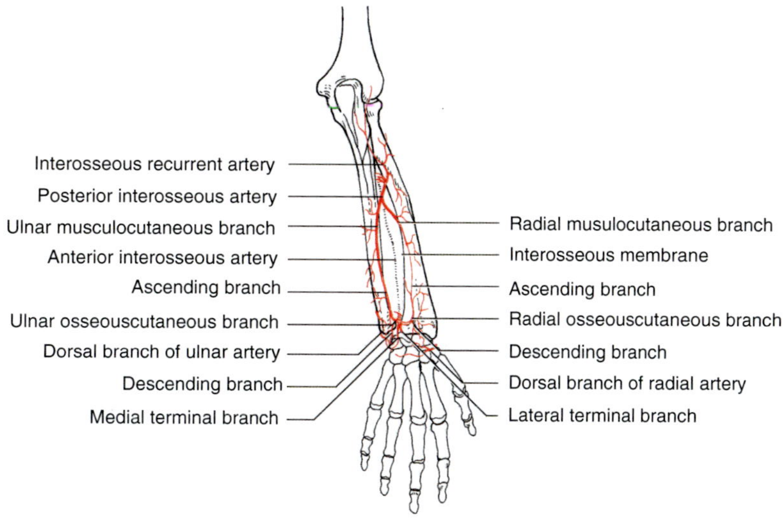

Fig. 12.1 Vascular anatomy of the posterior interosseous artery

C. Hou et al., *Surgical Atlas of Perforator Flaps: A Microsurgical Dissection Technique*,
DOI 10.1007/978-94-017-9834-1_12, © Springer Science+Business Media Dordrecht 2015

12.2 Illustrative Case

A 39-year-old man suffered a heat-press injury over his dorsum of the hand. The wound was extensive after debridement of the full-thickness eschar, measuring 11.0×7.0 cm (Fig. 12.2).

Flap Design

The flap was designed along the axis line between the extensor condyle of the humerus and the radial side of the ulnar head (Fig. 12.3) and centered around the perforating site preoperatively examined with a Doppler probe, usually 2.5 cm above the ulnar head (Fig. 12.4).

Flap Elevation

Firstly, the ulnar subcutaneous tissue of the flap was incised to the deep fascial surface, the flap was then raised above the deep fascia, then the perforator was identified and preserved. The whole flap was raised, keeping the interosseous artery intact in the deep septum. The cephalic vein was protected carefully in the radial side; the forearm posterior cutaneous nerve was exposed and kept intact (Fig. 12.5).

When the flap was separated at the middle-distal third of the forearm, attention was paid to the course of the perforating branches of the intermuscular septum. These perforating branches were kept to ensure the backflow of the flap (Fig. 12.6).

The extensor tendon, musculus extensor digiti minimi, and extensor carpi radialis muscle were freed, the perforating branches were separated intramuscularly up to the posterior interosseous vessel, the vessel pedicle was separated by long section, and the posterior interosseous nerve concomitant with the vessel was separated and protected.

The vessel pedicle was separated proximally and ligated up to the originating plane of interosseous membrane (Fig. 12.7).

Flap Transfer and Insetting

The flap is then rotated to its new position. The wrist was kept in extension and maintained in that position by using a metallic palmar splint for the duration of the flap healing (Fig. 12.8).

Follow-Up

Healing was complete and without complications. Functional and cosmetic results were excellent (Fig. 12.9).

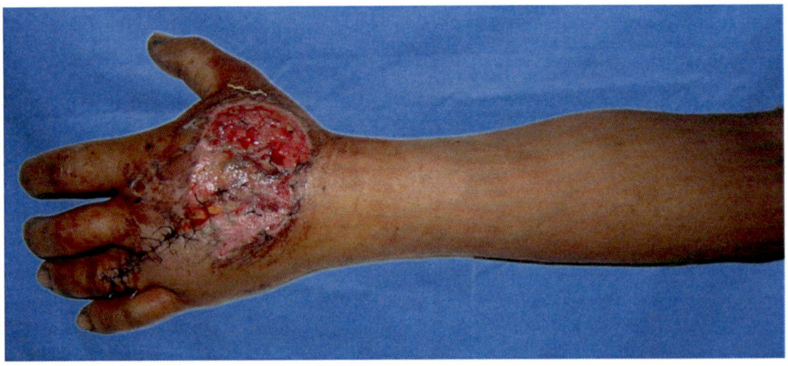

Fig. 12.2 Preoperative view

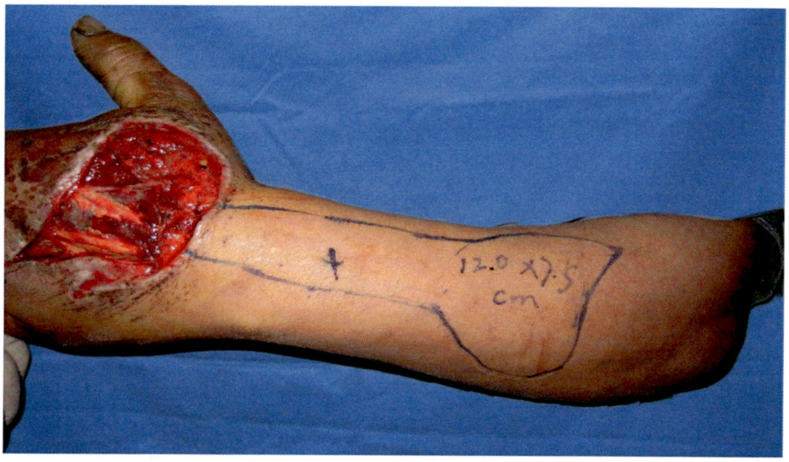

Fig. 12.3 Flap design

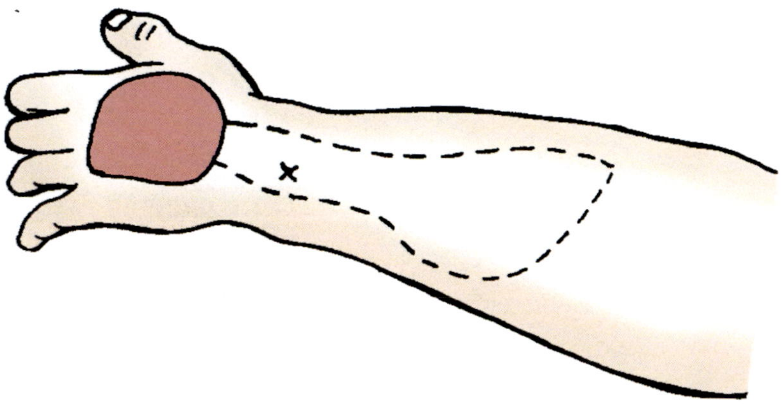

Fig. 12.4 Schematic drawing of flap design

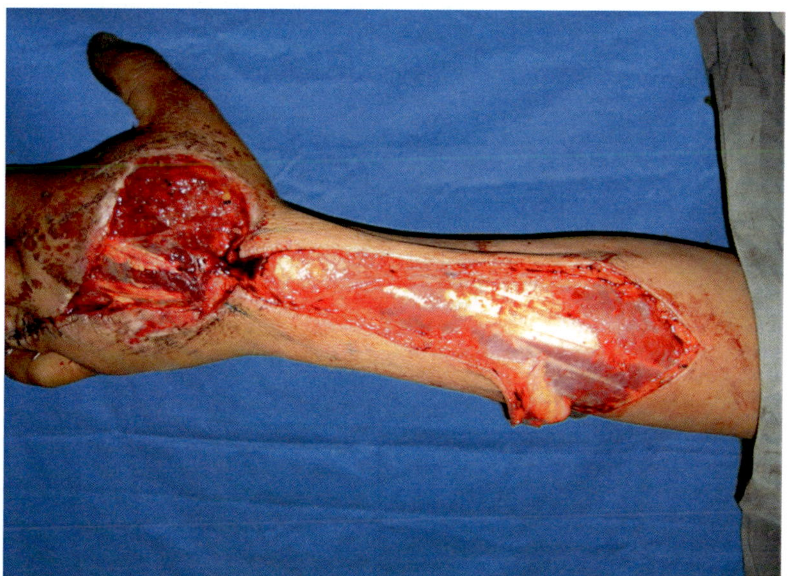

Fig. 12.5 Flap elevation

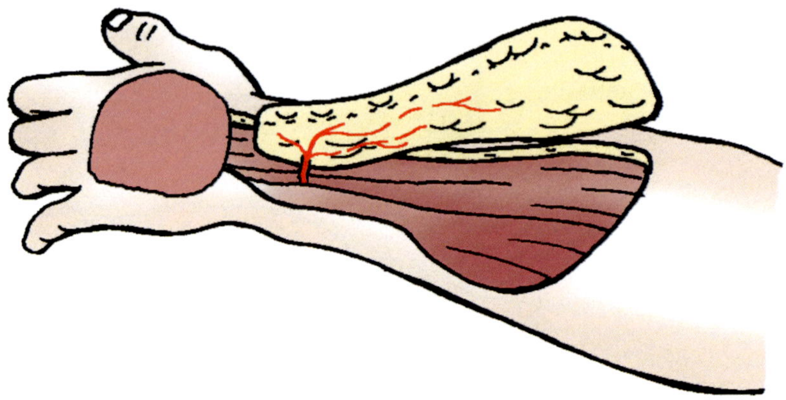

Fig. 12.6 Schematic drawing of the flap elevation

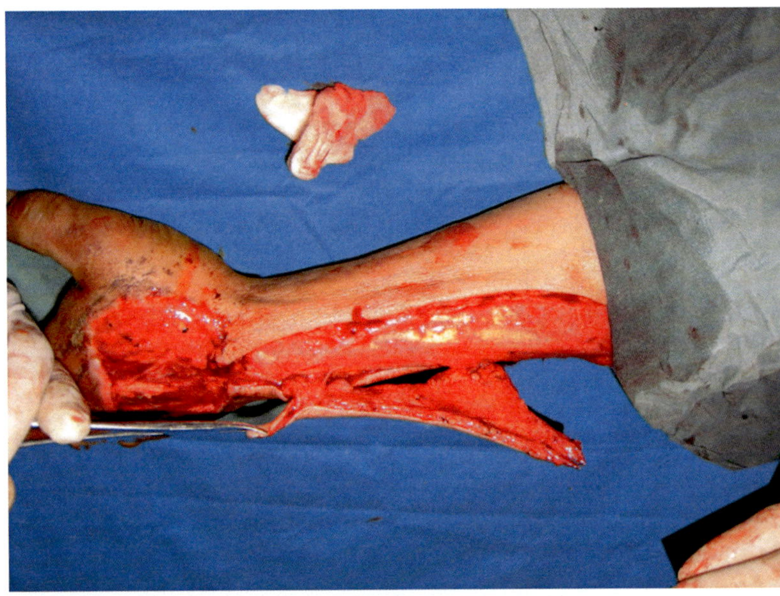

Fig. 12.7 The vessel pedicle was separated

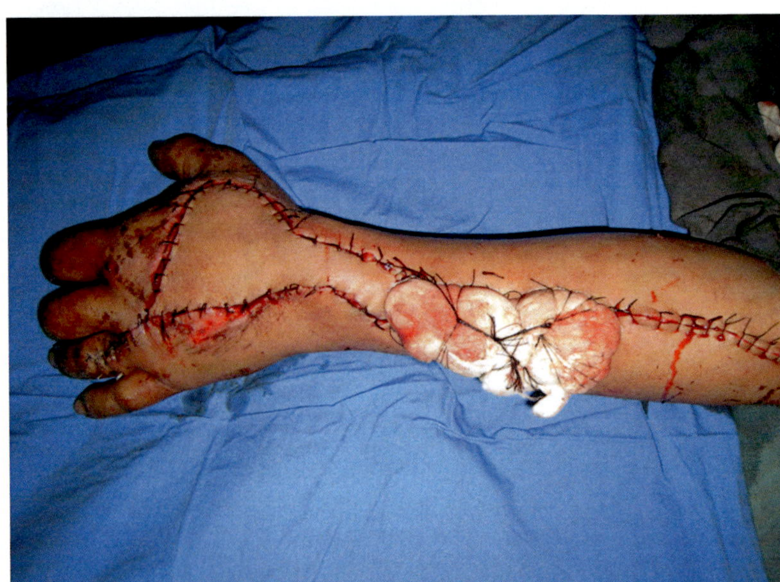

Fig. 12.8 Flap transfer and insetting

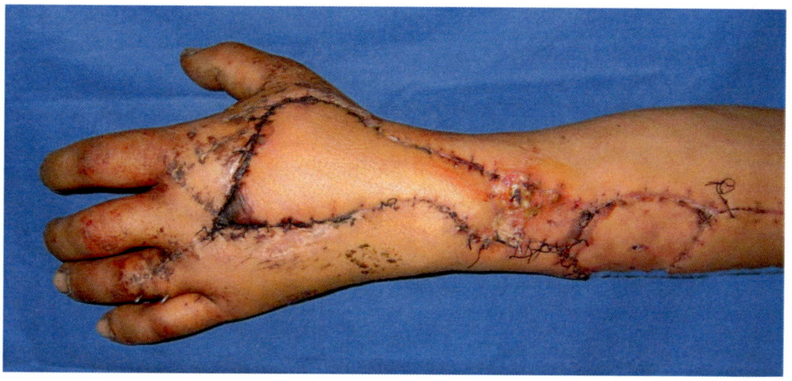

Fig. 12.9 Postoperative view

Pearls

The main advantages of the posterior interosseous perforator flap for hand coverage include its fineness, its excellent texture and color match, its easy accessibility, and its minimal donor-site morbidity [9–11].

Pitfalls

The posterior interosseous artery may become very small as it travels distally in approximately 6 % of the cases [5, 12].

Nerves crossing the arterial system may be managed with a neurotomy and immediate repair to regain near-normal muscle power.

To avoid problems related to the limited distal reach, one can base the flap on an exteriorized pedicle while maintaining the wrist in slight extension with a splint for 3 weeks.

References

1. Zancolli EA, Angrigiani C. Posterior interosseous island forearm flap. J Hand Surg Br. 1988;13(2):130–5.
2. Penteado CV, Masquelet AC, Chevrel JP. The anatomic basis of the fascio-cutaneous flap of the posterior interosseous artery. Surg Radiol Anat. 1986;8(4):209–15.
3. Sun C, Wang YL, Ding ZH, et al. Anatomical basis of a proximal fasciocutaneous extension of the distal-based posterior interosseous flap that allows exclusion of the proximal posterior interosseous artery. J Plast Reconstr Aesthet Surg. 2015;68:17–25.
4. Bayon P, Pho RW. Anatomical basis of dorsal forearm flap. Based on posterior interosseous vessels. J Hand Surg Br. 1988;13(4):435–9.
5. Buchler U, Frey HP. Retrograde posterior interosseous flap. J Hand Surg. 1991;16(2):283–92.
6. Costa H, Soutar DS. The distally based island posterior interosseous flap. Br J Plast Surg. 1988;41(3):221–7.
7. Angrigiani C, Grilli D, Dominikow D, Zancolli EA. Posterior interosseous reverse forearm flap: experience with 80 consecutive cases. Plast Reconstr Surg. 1993;92(2):285–93.
8. Costa H, Comba S, Martins A, Rodrigues J, Reis J, Amarante J. Further experience with the posterior interosseous flap. Br J Plast Surg. 1991;44(6):449–55.
9. Li KW, Liu J, Liu MJ, Xie SL, Liu CX. Free multilobed posterior interosseous artery perforator flap for multi-finger skin defect reconstruction. J Plast Reconstr Aesthet Surg. 2014;68:9–16.
10. Zhang YX, Qian Y, Pu Z, et al. Reverse bipaddle posterior interosseous artery perforator flap. Plast Reconstr Surg. 2013;131(4):552e–62.
11. Gong X, Lu LJ. Reconstruction of severe contracture of the first web space using the reverse posterior interosseous artery flap. J Trauma. 2011;71(6):1745–9.
12. Cheng MH, Chen HC, Santamaria E, et al. Preoperative ultrasound Doppler study and clinical correlation of free posterior interosseous flap. Changgeng Yi Xue Za Zhi. 1997;20(4):258–64.

13 Posterolateral Mid-Forearm Perforator Flap

Zheng and Lin reported the anatomical basis and clinical application of posterolateral mid-forearm perforator flap [1, 2].

13.1 Vascular Anatomy

Three patterns of the perforator were observed in the posterolateral aspect of the mid-forearm [3].

In pattern I, the perforator was the lateral terminal branch of the posterior interosseous artery that traveled initially between the contiguous border of supinator and abductor pollicis longus and gave off several muscular branches to the surrounding muscles along its course; the trunk of this perforator continued to emerge superficially at the septum between the extensor digitorum and extensor carpi radialis brevis and pierced the deep fascia at the posterolateral aspect of the mid-forearm. It pierced the deep fascia at the site 12.5 ± 0.3 cm inferior to the lateral humeral epicondyle along the line between the lateral humeral epicondyle and the radial head (Fig. 13.1).

In pattern II, the perforator originated from the proximal segment of the radial artery or the radial recurrent artery. It run initially at the septum between pronator teres and supinator in close contact with the radial periosteum and gave off several minute periosteal branches to nourish the middle segment of the radius. The trunk of this perforator traveled downward through the septum between extensor digitorum and extensor carpi radialis brevis and pierced the deep fascia at the posterolateral aspect of the mid-forearm. It pierced the deep fascia at the site 11.8 ± 0.2 cm inferior to the lateral humeral epicondyle along the line between the lateral humeral epicondyle and the radial head [4].

In pattern III, the perforator originated from the middle segment of the radial artery. It traveled obliquely downward along the inferior margin of pronator teres or traversed across the insertion of pronator teres, giving off several periosteal branches to form a vascular network in the mid-to-distal segment of the radius. The trunk of this perforator emerged superficially through the septum between extensor digitorum and extensor carpi radialis brevis, piecing the deep fascia at the posterolateral aspect of the mid-forearm. It pierced the deep fascia at the site 15.8 ± 0.4 cm inferior to the lateral humeral epicondyle along the line between the lateral humeral epicondyle and the radial head.

C. Hou et al., *Surgical Atlas of Perforator Flaps: A Microsurgical Dissection Technique*,
DOI 10.1007/978-94-017-9834-1_13, © Springer Science+Business Media Dordrecht 2015

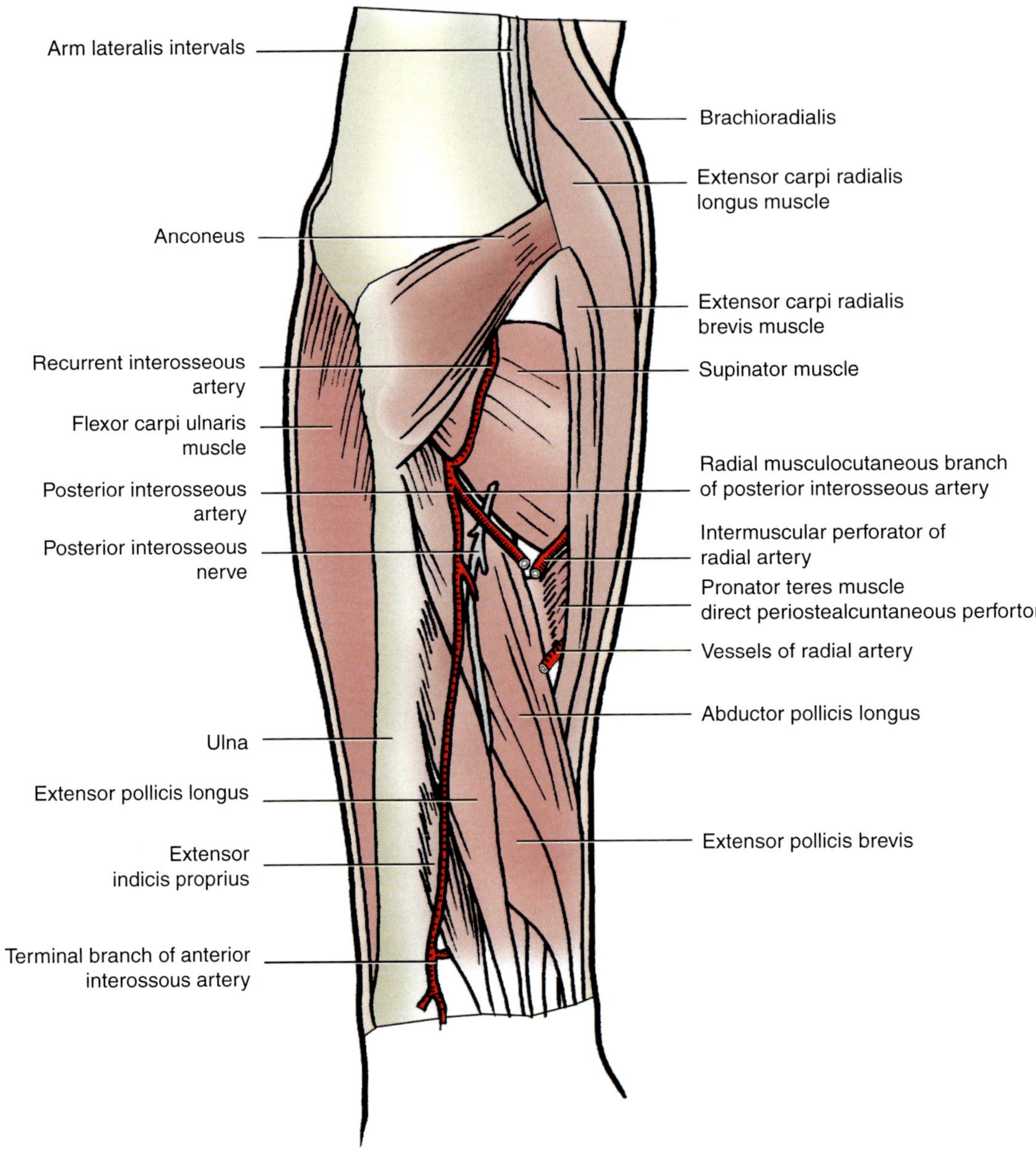

Fig. 13.1 Vascular anatomy of the posterolateral mid-forearm perforator flap

13.2 Illustrative Case

A 64-year-old male patient sustained a strangulation injury from a drilling machine at the forearm and wrist, leading to fractures of the radius and ulna, a soft tissue defect of 8.5×4.0 cm in size over the dorsal aspect of the mid-to-distal forearm.

The patient underwent plate and screw fixation for fractures of the radius and ulna; reconstruction of the avulsed tendons, nerves, and vessels; reattachment of the degloved skin; as well as application of the vacuum suction device at the dorsal defect of the forearm in emergency surgery (Fig. 13.2).

Flap Design (Fig. 13.3)

Ten days later, the posterolateral mid-forearm perforator flap with a size of 10.5×4.5 cm was designed (Fig. 13.4).

Flap Elevation

A tourniquet was used on the affected arm without exsanguination. Handheld Doppler probe was employed to locate the surface position of the perforator at the posterolateral aspect of the forearm 12.5–15.8 cm inferior to the lateral humeral epicondyle. The line between the lateral humeral epicondyle and the radial styloid process was defined as the axial line with the forearm in neutral posture.

The template of the flap was then outlined on the posterolateral aspect of the forearm with the dimension ranging up to 1 cm larger than the defect size. An incision was first made at the anterior margin of the template and was gradually extended backward at the subfascial layer.

When the septum between extensor digitorum and extensor carpi radialis brevis was exposed, the perforator was identified by its engorged venae comitantes and carefully protected. Incision was continued along the perimeter of the template, ligating, and dividing the minute vessels encountered as well as both ends of the lateral branch of the posterior antebrachial cutaneous nerve and its accompanying veins (Fig. 13.5). Isolation was performed around the perforator to obtain a vascular bundle of 1–2 cm in length. It was unnecessary to trace the perforator to its source artery whenever a pedicled perforator flap was planned to cover the defect. Consequently, the source artery of the perforator adopted was not known in the operation (Fig. 13.6).

Flap Transfer

The flap was harvested and transferred to cover the defect, and the donor site was covered with a split-thickness skin graft (Fig. 13.7).

Follow-Up

The flap survived completely and the skin graft took well.

The patient was followed up for 7 months and had a full function restoration of the repaired arm (Fig. 13.8).

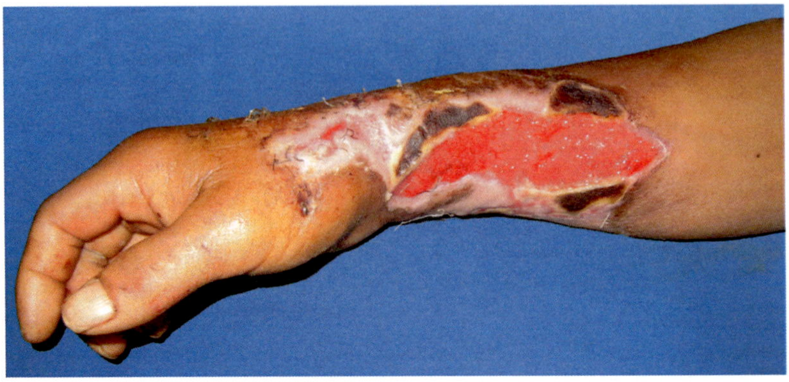

Fig. 13.2 Preoperative view

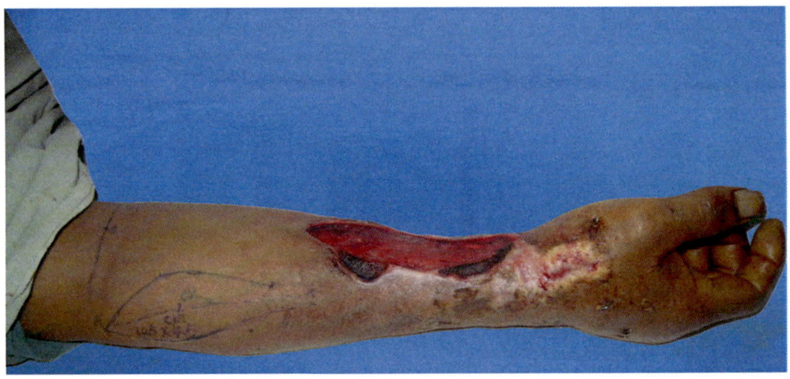

Fig. 13.3 Flap design

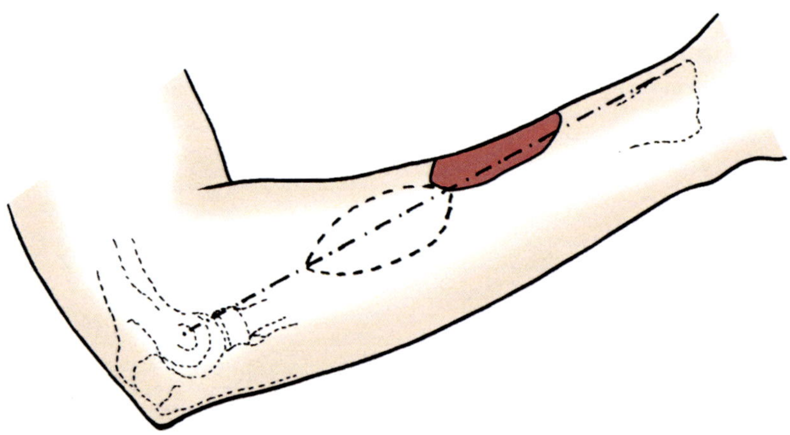

Fig. 13.4 Schematic drawing of the flap design

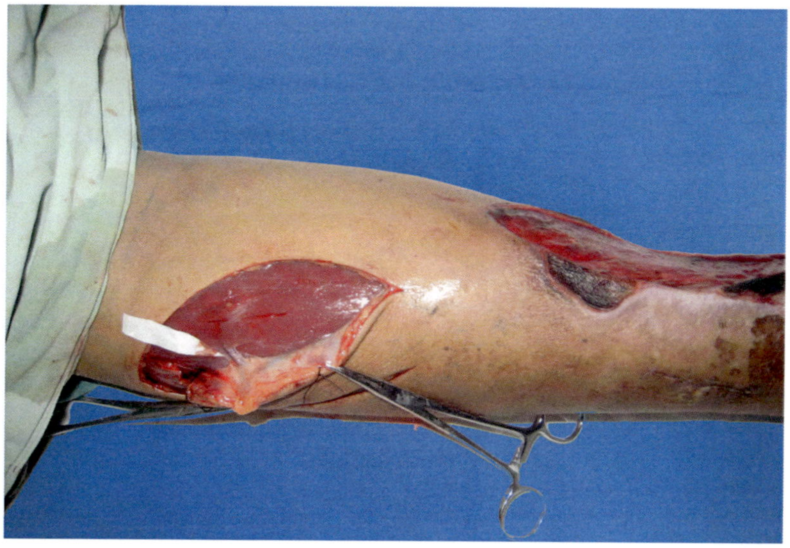

Fig. 13.5 Perforator vessel visualization

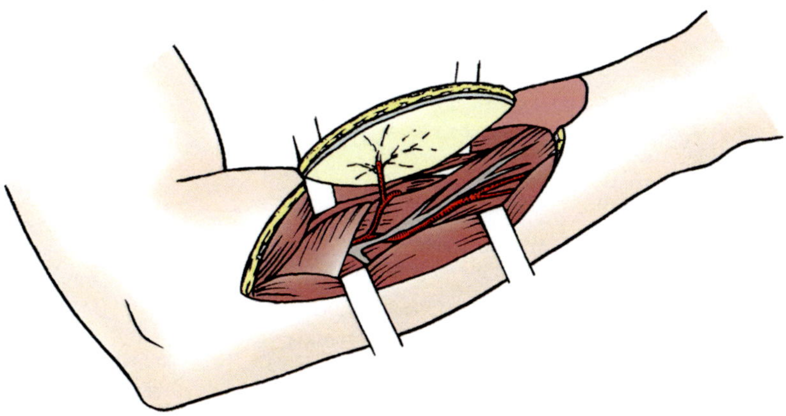

Fig. 13.6 Schematic drawing of the flap elevation

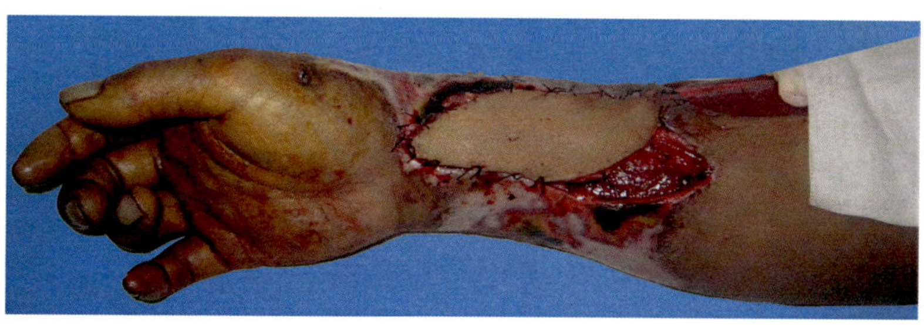

Fig. 13.7 Postoperative view

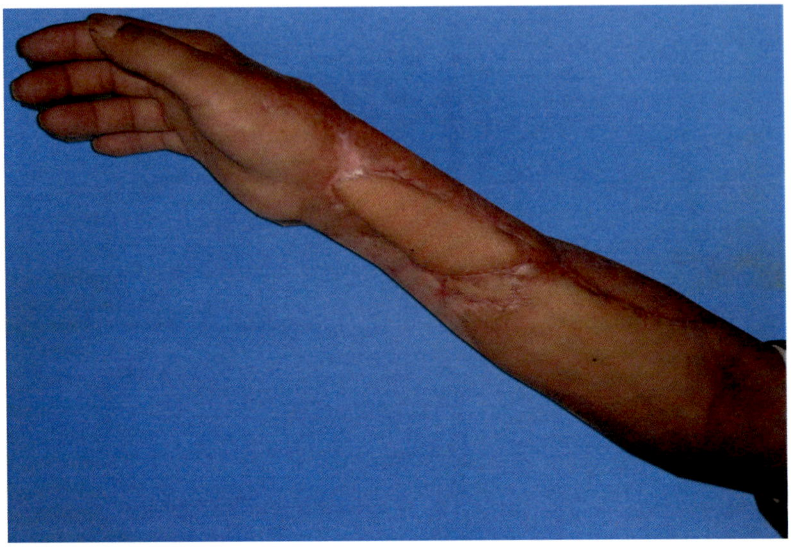

Fig. 13.8 Follow-up

Pearls

The perforator flap can be harvested without major jeopardy to the vascularization of the hand [5].

The location of the perforator was often adjacent to the proximal margin of the wound, indicating that not long pedicle are necessary and thus no reverse intramuscular dissection is required, which together make this method particularly suitable and convenient for coverage of small- to medium-sized tissue defects in the distal one-third of the forearm with minimal trauma [6].

Pitfalls

The forearm has the function of rotation; there is a relatively large degree of mobility between the skin and the underlying deep fascia; hence, when drawing the template, the forearm is recommended to be held in the neutral posture for accuracy of locating the perforator.

References

1. Zhuang YH, Lin J, Fu FH, Cai ZD, Huang HM, Zheng HP. The posterolateral mid-forearm perforator flap: anatomical study and clinical application. Microsurgery. 2013;18(4):78–81.
2. Lin J, Yu YL, Zheng HP. Perforator flap in the middle segment of posterolateral forearm for dorsal defects at the lower forearm. Zhonghua Zheng Xing Wai Ke Za Zhi. 2012;28(5):325–8.
3. Mei J, Morris SF, Ji W, Li H, Zhou R, Tang M. An anatomic study of the dorsal forearm perforator flaps. Surg Radiol Anat. 2013;35(8):695–700.
4. Ding YC. Micro-anatomy of nutrient vessels of skin of dorsal surface of forearm and its clinical applications. Zhonghua Zheng Xing Shao Shang Wai Ke Za Zhi. 1989;5(1):36–9, 77–38.
5. Yang D, Tang M. Clinical application of perforator flap in repairing soft tissue defects of extremities. Zhongguo Xiu Fu Chong Jian Wai Ke Za Zhi. 2011;25(9):1047–50.
6. Liu DX, Wang H, Li XD, Du SX. Three kinds of forearm flaps for hand skin defects: experience of 65 cases. Arch Orthop Trauma Surg. 2011;131(5):675–80.

Dorsal Metacarpal Artery Perforator Flaps

14

The first dorsal metacarpal artery (FDMA) flap (kite flap) was firstly described by Foucher and Braun [1].

As firstly described by Quaba and Davison [2], the DMA (dorsal metacarpal artery) flap can be harvested without incorporating the DMA [3]. This flap is based on cutaneous perforators originating from the DMAs.

This flap does not include the DMA, and its vascular supply is based solely on the cutaneous perforator emanating either directly from the DMA or from the communicating branch between the DMA and the palmar metacarpal artery.

14.1 Vascular Anatomy

The blood supply to the dorsal skin of the hand and digits is provided by (1) the DMAs, which vascularize the proximal portion of the hand, and (2) the dorsal perforating metacarpal arterial branches from the deep palmar arch, which supply the distal hand and proximal phalanx [4]. These two major arterial systems form the basis for direct and reverse DMA flaps (Fig. 14.1).

The cutaneous perforator is very reliable and can almost always be found within the second through the fourth intermetacarpal spaces roughly 1 cm proximal to the metacarpal neck. This is in sharp contrast to the third and fourth DMAs, which can sometimes be absent.

The FDMA originated from the radial artery or the dorsalis superficialis antebrachialis artery. There are vascular connections between the dorsal digital branches of the second through fourth DMA arteries and the dorsal branches of the PPD arteries. These connections make it possible to harvest an extended reverse DMA flap based on retrograde flow from the dorsal branches of the PPD artery.

The second dorsal metacarpal artery (SDMA) generally runs along a line joining the anatomic snuffbox and second webspace. The SDMA originated from the dorsal carpal arch or the deep palmar arch, the FDMA, the anterior interosseous artery, or the radial artery [5].

C. Hou et al., *Surgical Atlas of Perforator Flaps: A Microsurgical Dissection Technique*,
DOI 10.1007/978-94-017-9834-1_14,

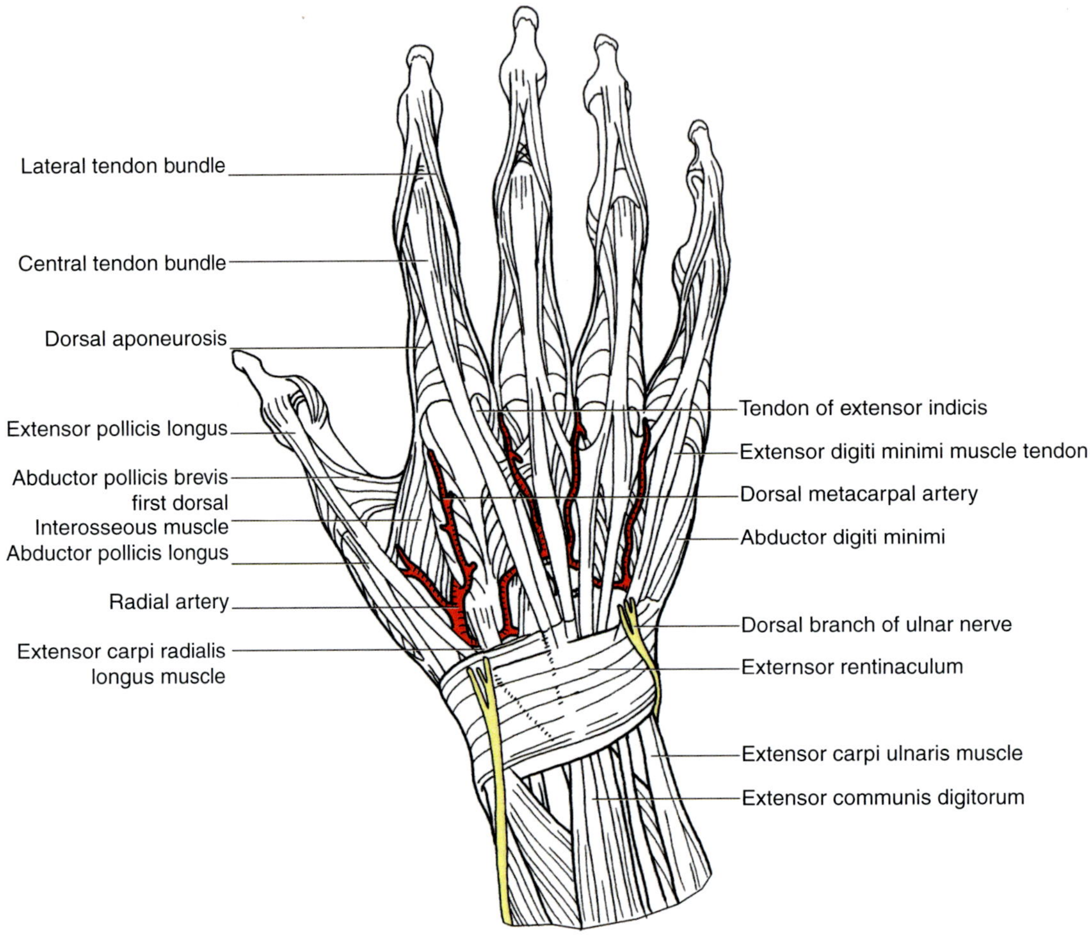

Fig. 14.1 Vascular anatomy of the first dorsal metacarpal artery

14.2 Illustrative Case

Case 1

This 18-year-old man was operated on using this procedure. He sustained a work-related injury. The index finger was involved, and the skin defect was located over the proximal interphalangeal (PIP) joint (Fig. 14.2).

Flap Design

The reverse FDMA flap is designed over the dorsum of the first metacarpal bone along the mid radial line of the index finger.

Once a cutaneous perforator has been identified, it can be confirmed with handheld pencil Doppler device.

The dorsal cutaneous perforator of the DMA is located just distal to the juncture of tendons and roughly 0.5–1 cm proximal to the metacarpal neck within the intermetacarpal space (Fig. 14.3). The flap axis is designed parallel to the long axis of the metacarpal (Fig. 14.4).

Flap Elevation

Elevation of the FDMA flap begins distally by incising the flap outline over the dorsal proximal metacarpal bone in a proximal to distal direction, just above the peritenon layer. The perforator flap is raised subdermally to develop a subcutaneous pedicle (Fig. 14.5).

The flap is elevated from proximal to distal until the juncturae tendinae is reached.

At this point, the more distal portion of the skin flap is elevated off the surrounding subcutaneous tissue, and subcutaneous tissue and fascia surrounding the perforator are freed until adequate rotation is possible without any excessive twisting or tension on the perforator (Fig. 14.6).

Flap Transfer

The perforator pedicle is seen with a perivascular soft tissue cuff. The flap is elevated and transferred to the palmar index finger defect (Fig. 14.7).

Flap Insetting

The flap is inset into the defect, and the donor site is covered with a full-thickness skin graft (Fig. 14.8).

Follow-Up

The flap survived smoothly (Fig. 14.9).

Case 2

In this 32-year-old man the defect resulted from a crush injury. Radial dorsum defect after index digital avulsion injury with exposed extensor apparatus over the distal and middle phalanges and the PIP joint and the dorsum defect after thumb avulsion injury with exposed extensor apparatus over the distal phalange are shown in Fig. 14.10.

The reverse radial dorsal digital artery perforator flap is designed on the radial dorsum aspect of the first metacarpal area.

The reverse first dorsal metacarpal artery perforator flap is designed over the dorsum of the second metacarpal bone along the mid radial line of the middle finger (Fig. 14.11).

Flap Elevation

The flap is elevated from proximal to distal until the juncturae tendinae is reached (Fig. 14.12).

Flap Insetting

The flap is inset into the defect, and the donor site is covered with a full-thickness skin graft (Fig. 14.13).

The flap survived smoothly (Fig. 14.14).

Case 3

A 27-year-old man suffered circular saw injury to his ring finger. Radial dorsum defect after ring avulsion injury with exposed extensor apparatus over the proximal and middle phalanges and the PIP joint. The reverse FDMA flap is designed over the dorsum of the fourth metacarpal bone along the mid radial line of the ring finger. The flap was harvested from the third interdigital space (Fig. 14.15).

Flap Design (Fig. 14.16)

The reverse first dorsal metacarpal artery perforator flap is designed over the dorsum of the second metacarpal bone along the mid radial line of the middle finger (Fig. 14.17).

Flap Elevation (Fig. 14.18)

The flap is elevated from proximal to distal until the juncturae tendinae is reached (Fig. 14.19).

Flap Insetting

The flap is inset into the defect, and the donor site is closed directly (Fig. 14.20).

The flap survived smoothly (Fig. 14.21).

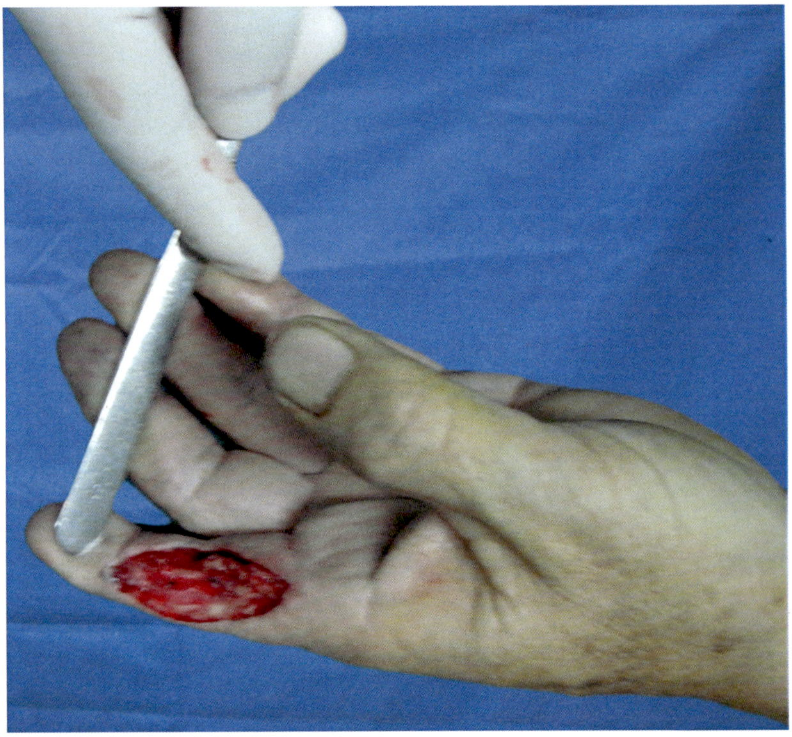

Fig. 14.2 Preoperative view

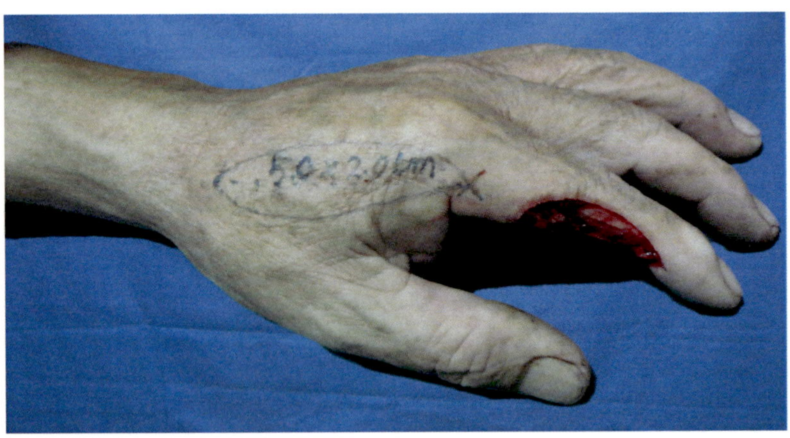

Fig. 14.3 Flap design

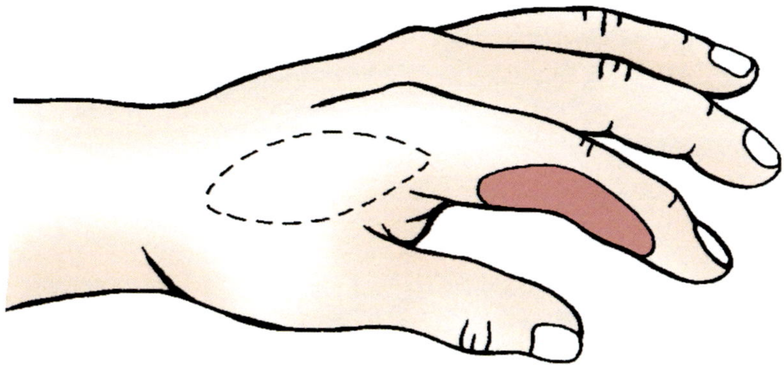

Fig. 14.4 Schematic drawing of the flap design

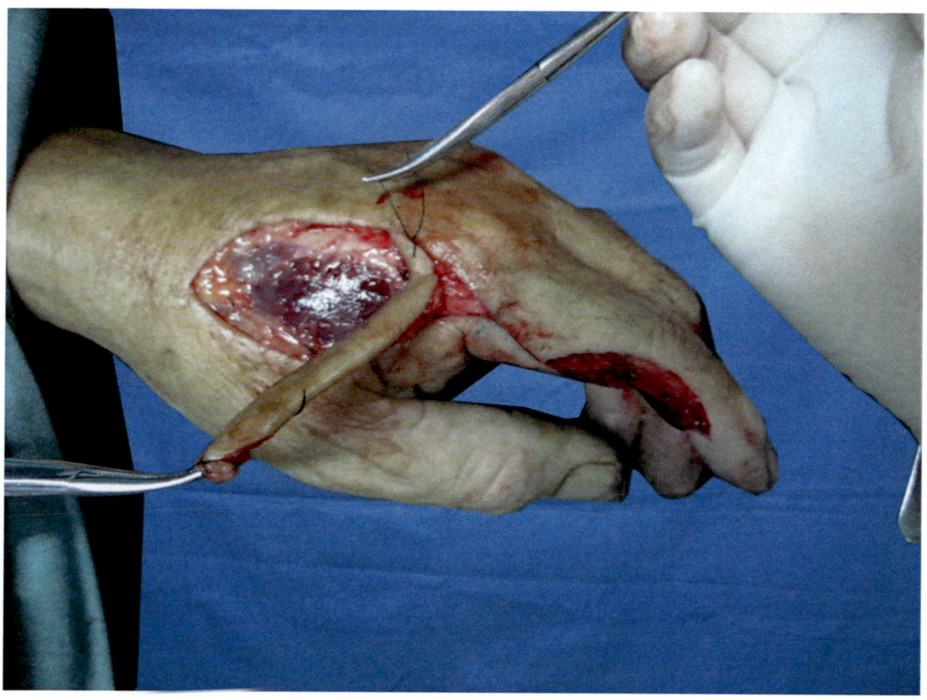

Fig. 14.5 Flap elevation

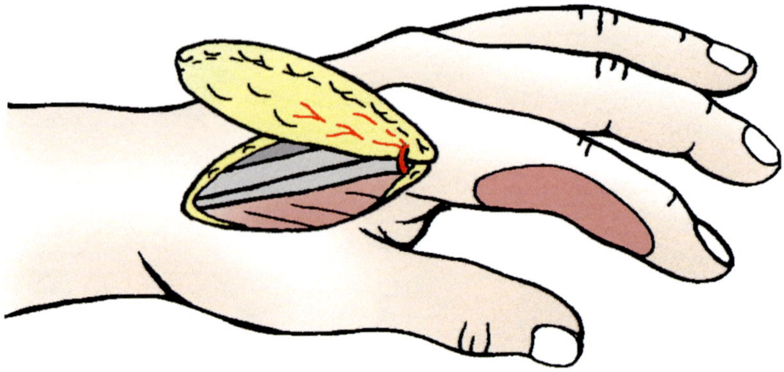

Fig. 14.6 Schematic drawing of the flap elevation

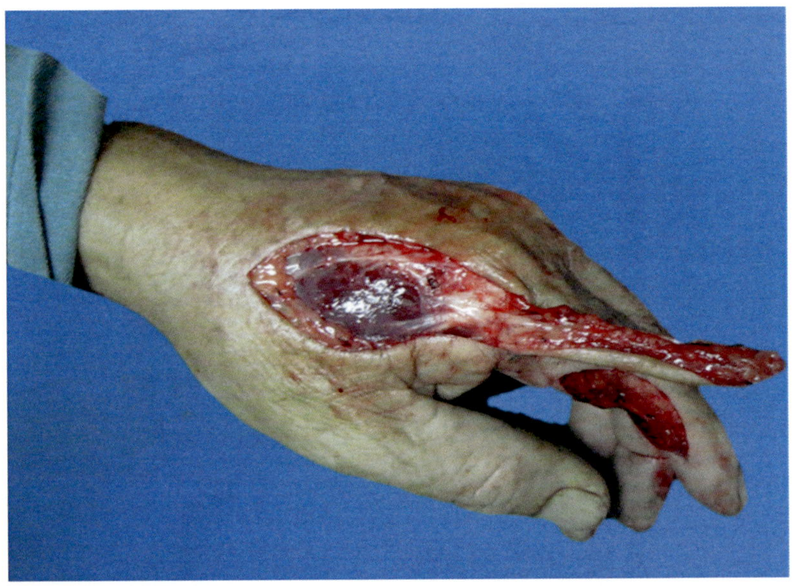

Fig. 14.7 Flap rotation

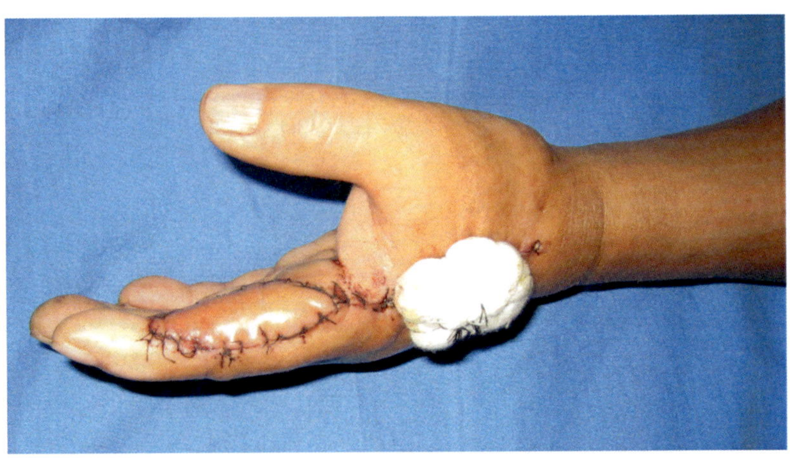

Fig. 14.8 Flap insetting

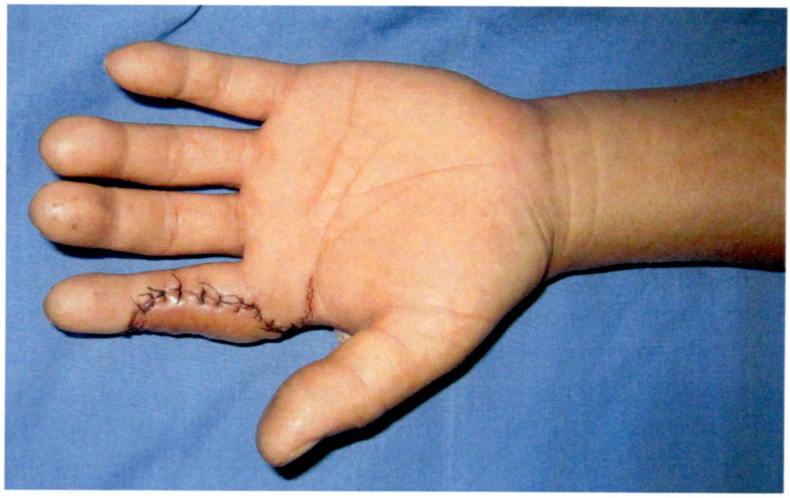

Fig. 14.9 Postoperative view

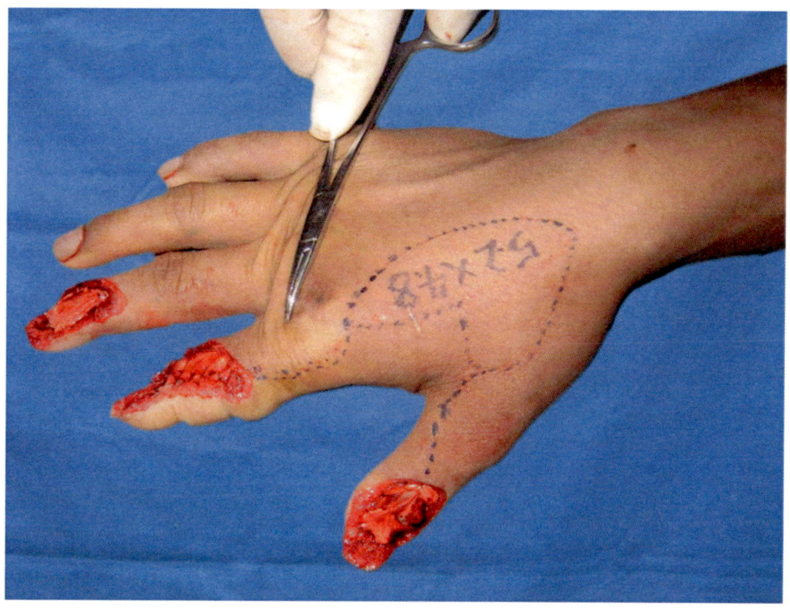

Fig. 14.10 Preoperative view

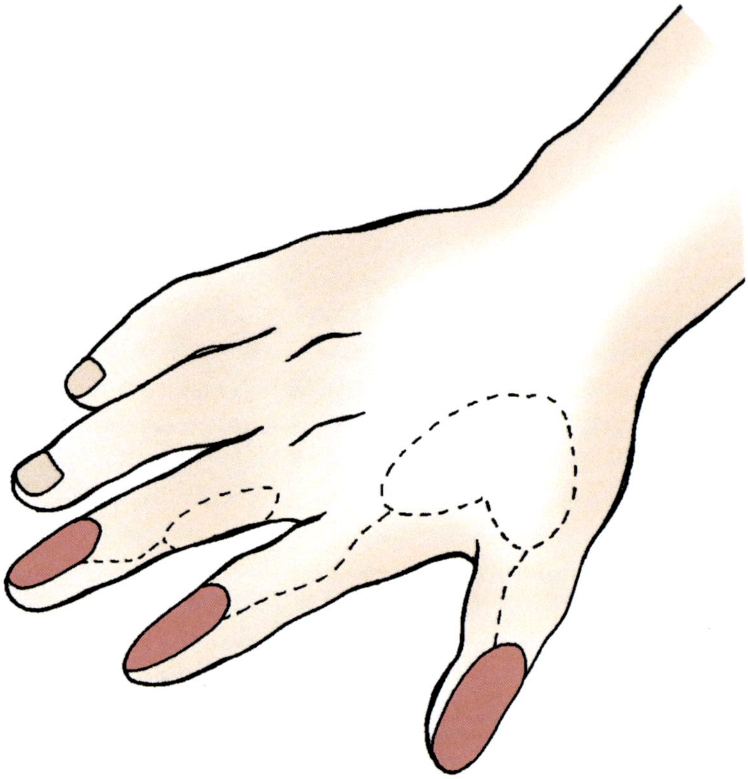

Fig. 14.11 Schematic drawing of the flap design

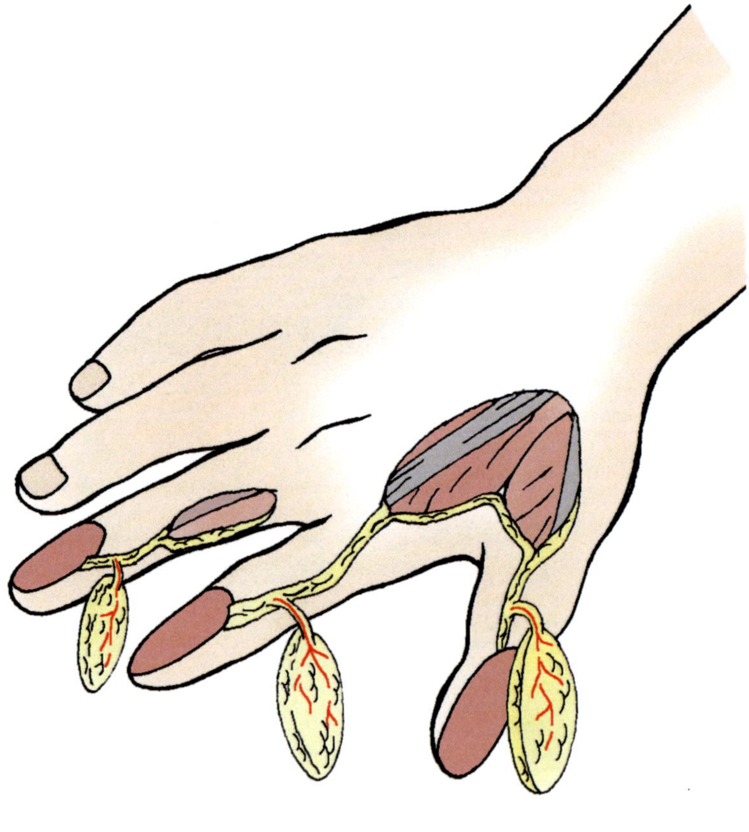

Fig. 14.12 Flap elevation

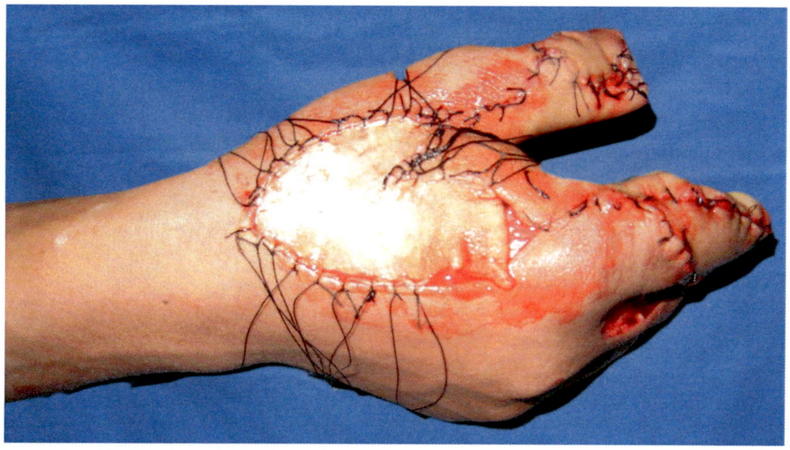

Fig. 14.13 Flap insetting

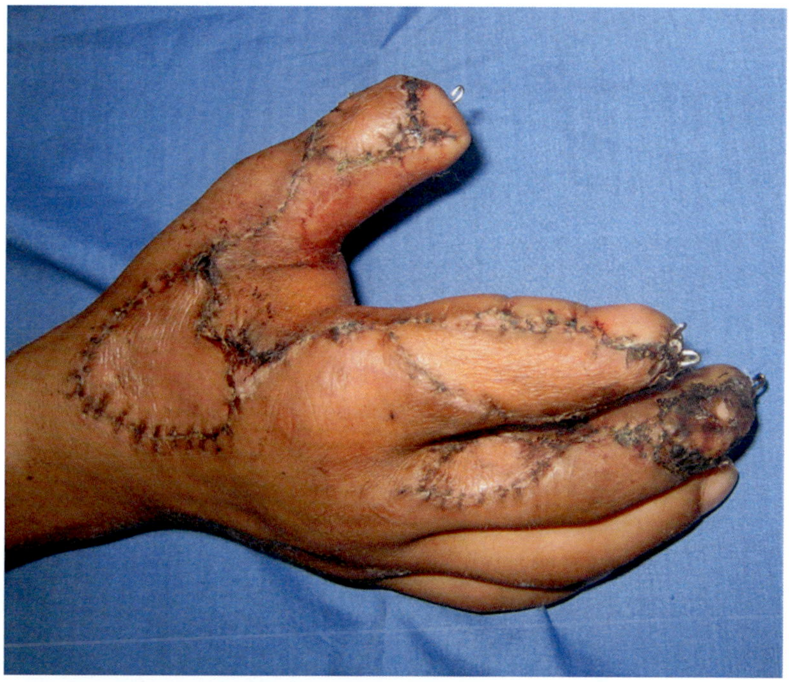

Fig. 14.14 Postoperative view

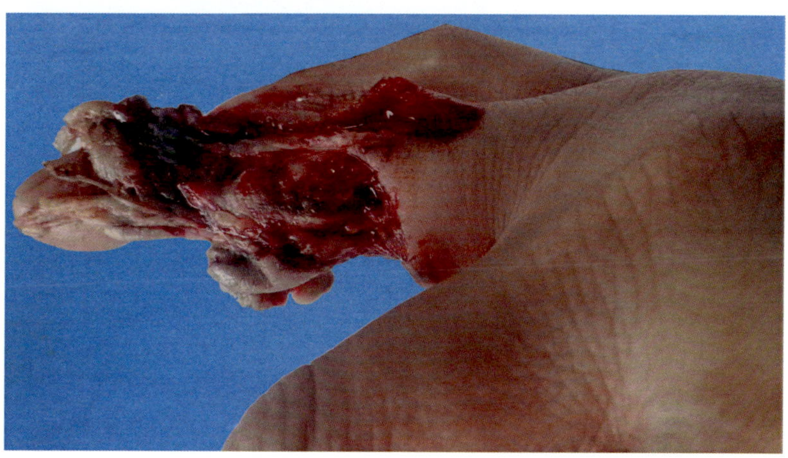

Fig. 14.15 Preoperative view

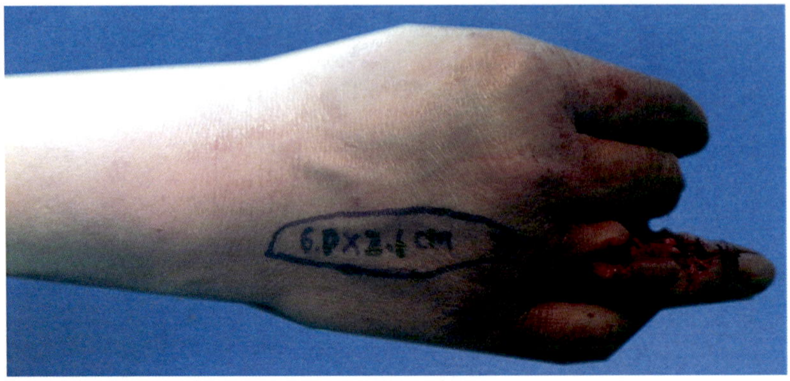

Fig. 14.16 Flap design

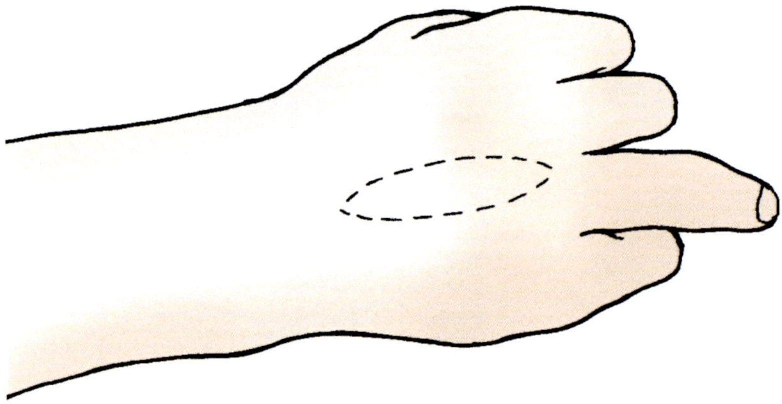

Fig. 14.17 Schematic drawing of the flap design

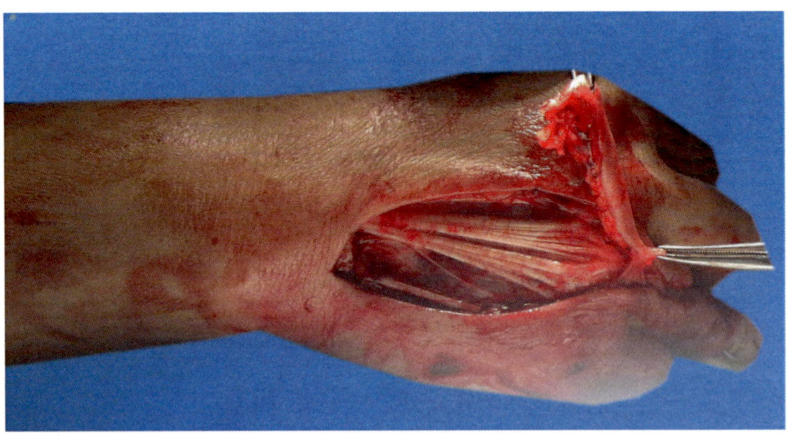

Fig. 14.18 Flap elevation

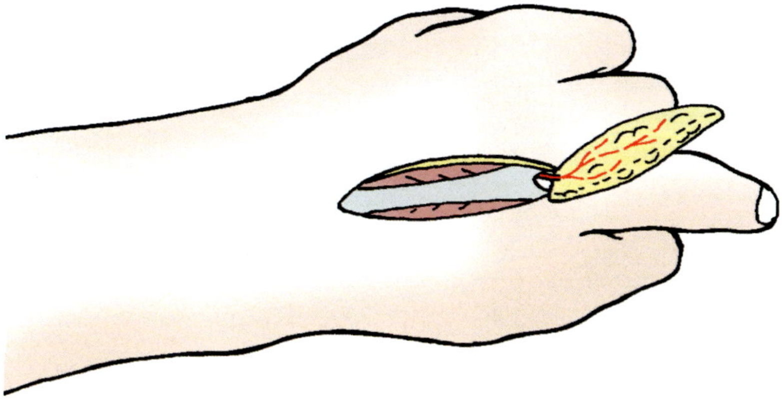

Fig. 14.19 Schematic drawing of the flap elevation and rotation

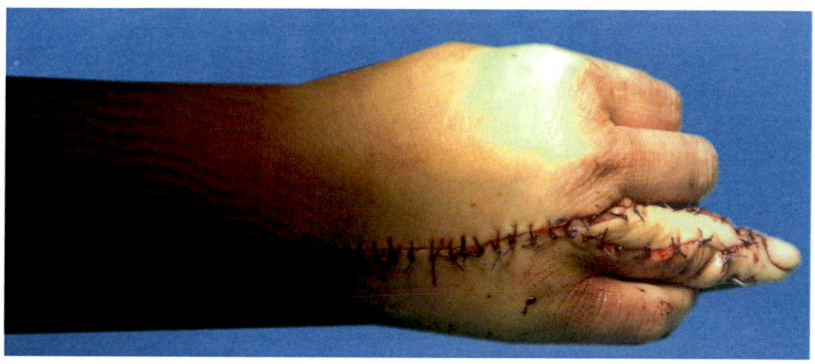

Fig. 14.20 Flap transfer

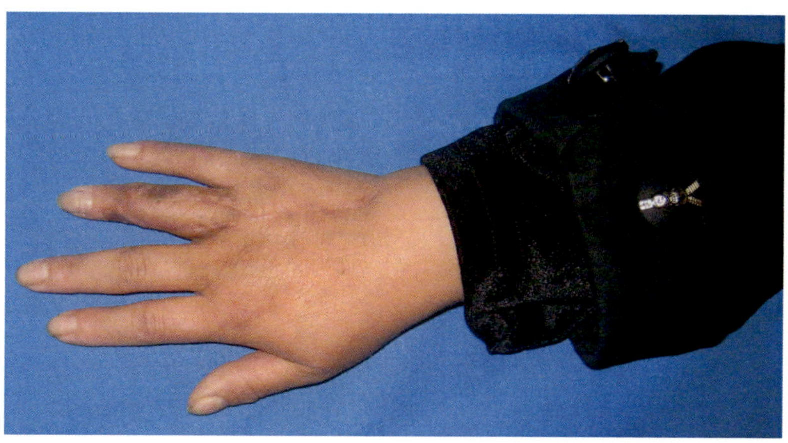

Fig. 14.21 Postoperative view

Pearls

The advantages of this perforator-based DMA flap include ease of elevation and thinner coverage for dorsal digital defects.

Pitfalls

The FDMA lies just superficial to the first dorsal interosseous fascia, necessitating inclusion of the latter during flap elevation to prevent damage to the pedicle [6].

The pedicle should not be skeletonized and should be raised with a generous cuff of fibrofatty tissue [7].

If required, tunneling is performed by undermining the dorsal subcutaneous tissue and skin, and the flap is transferred into the defect without tension, compression, or kinking.

Flap insetting should be done with minimal tension and the least amount of sutures possible to accommodate postoperative swelling.

References

1. Foucher G, Braun JB. A new island flap transfer from the dorsum of the index to the thumb. Plast Reconstr Surg. 1979;63(3):344–9.
2. Quaba AA, Davison PM. The distally-based dorsal hand flap. Br J Plast Surg. 1990;43(1):28–39.
3. Sebastin SJ, Mendoza RT, Chong AK, et al. Application of the dorsal metacarpal artery perforator flap for resurfacing soft-tissue defects proximal to the fingertip. Plast Reconstr Surg. 2011;128(3):166e–78.
4. Yang D, Morris SF. Vascular basis of dorsal digital and metacarpal skin flaps. J Hand Surg. 2001;26(1):142–6.
5. Earley MJ, Milner RH. Dorsal metacarpal flaps. Br J Plast Surg. 1987;40(4):333–41.
6. Sherif MM. First dorsal metacarpal artery flap in hand reconstruction. II. Clinical application. J Hand Surg. 1994;19(1):32–8.
7. Zhang X, Shao X, Ren C, Wen S, Zhu H, Sun J. Coverage of dorsal-ulnar hand wounds with a reverse second dorsal metacarpal artery flap. J Reconstr Microsurg. 2012;28(3):167–73.

15 Dorso-ulnar Metacarpal Perforator Flap of the Little Finger

In hand surgery, several vascular pedicled island flaps taken from the dorsal skin of the hand and forearm are available for reconstruction of hands and fingers [1–4].

15.1 Vascular Anatomy

The dorsal branch of the ulnar artery branched from the ulnar artery approximately 3 cm from the styloid process of the ulna and passed dorsally under the flexor carpi ulnaris muscle. After giving off muscular and osseous branches to the flexor carpi ulnaris muscle and the pisiform bone, two cutaneous ascending and descending branches followed the fascial layer of the flexor carpi ulnaris muscle longitudinally (Fig. 15.1).

After it had given off a branch that contributed to the dorsal carpal arch, a descending branch of the dorsal ulnar artery coursed to the radial and ulnar sides of the fifth metacarpal. The ulnar branch had numerous microvascular connections to the underlying fascia of the hypothenar muscle. The mean arterial diameter of this branch (at a site branching to the dorsal carpal arch) was 0.5 mm. This descending branch gave off two to four skin perforators between the ulnar styloid and the fifth metacarpal and supplied the ulnar aspect of the dorsal wrist, where it was located over the sixth compartment of the extensor retinaculum. Communications from the dorsal branch of the ulnar artery to the palmar arterial system at the fifth metacarpal head were present in all specimens.

The venous drainage of the radial and ulnar aspects of the dorsum of the wrist was partly from the concomitant veins of the neurocutaneous perforating arteries from the dorsal branches of the radial and ulnar arteries and partly from the subcutaneous cephalic and basilic venous system.

C. Hou et al., *Surgical Atlas of Perforator Flaps: A Microsurgical Dissection Technique*,
DOI 10.1007/978-94-017-9834-1_15, © Springer Science+Business Media Dordrecht 2015

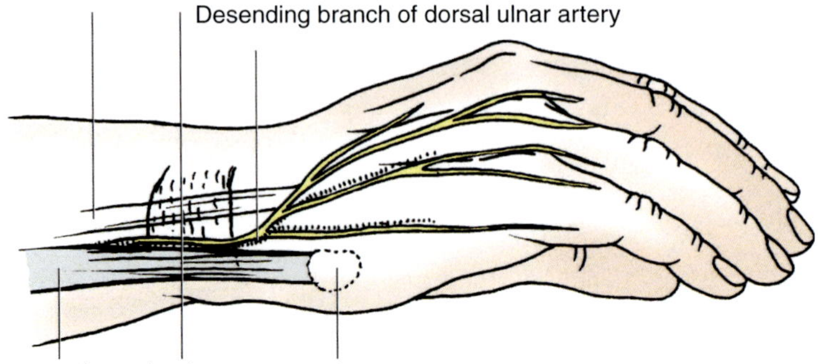

Fig. 15.1 Vascular anatomy of the dorsal branch of the ulnar artery

15.2 Illustrative Case

A 25-year-old man sustained a crush amputation to his middle and ring finger by a machine. Replantation was impossible, and the palmar site of little finger was necrotized. Because he wished to keep the little finger as long as possible, the flap procedure was planned for coverage of its exposed bone and tendon (Fig. 15.2).

Flap Design

The flap is designed over the distal half of the ulnar aspect of the hypothenar eminence (Fig. 15.3). This fasciocutaneous area is supplied by multiple perforating arteries from the ulnar palmar digital artery (UPDA) of the little finger. The pivot point (PP) of the reverse flap is located at the proximal phalangeal level. Sensory innervation of the area is chiefly provided by the dorsal branch of the ulnar nerve (DUN) (Fig. 15.4).

Flap Elevation (Fig. 15.5)

Flap dissection is performed in the subfascial plane from the dorsal side of the hand, and multiple perforating branches running transversely and arising from the ulnar palmar digital artery are identified and included in the flap (Fig. 15.6).

Flap Transfer

Communications of the dorsal branch of the ulnar artery with the palmar arterial system at the fifth metacarpal head were seen and preserved (Fig. 15.7).

Flap Insetting

The flap was rotated 180° to cover the defect (Fig. 15.8).

Follow-Up

The flap survived smoothly (Fig. 15.9).

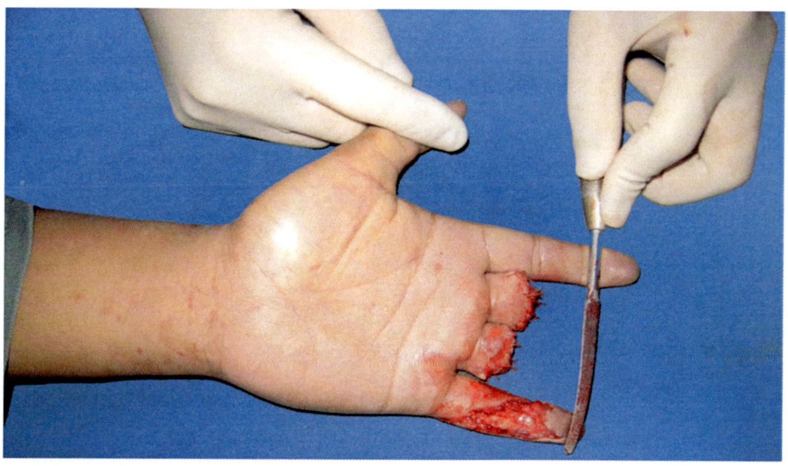

Fig. 15.2 Preoperative view

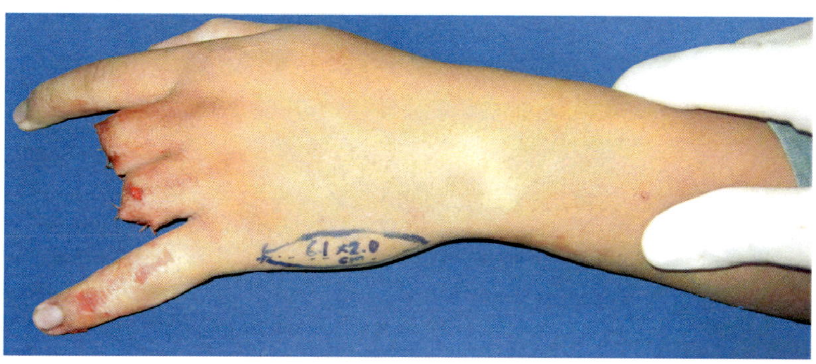

Fig. 15.3 Flap design

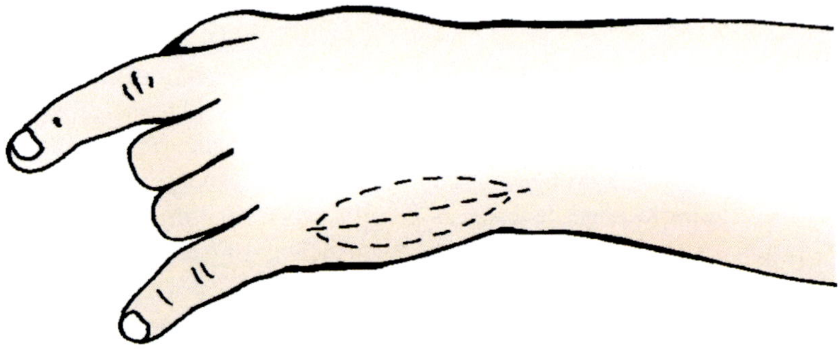

Fig. 15.4 Schematic drawing of the flap design

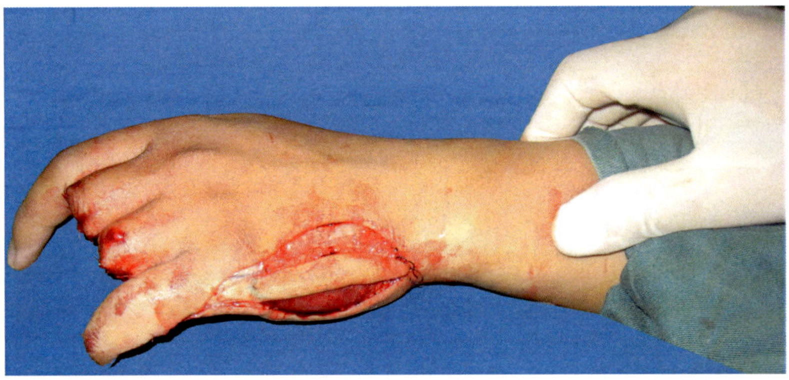

Fig. 15.5 Flap elevation

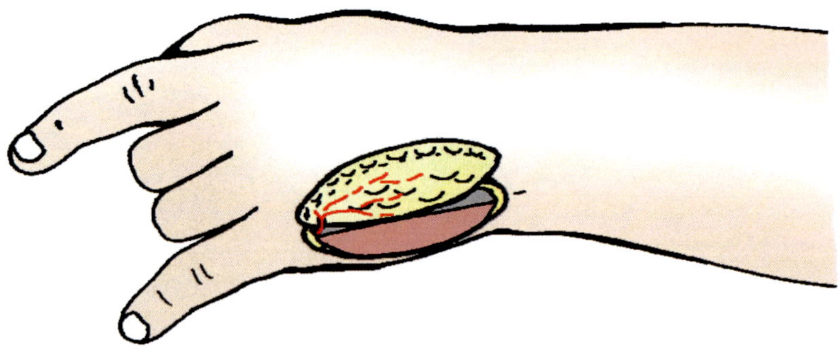

Fig. 15.6 Schematic drawing of the flap elevation

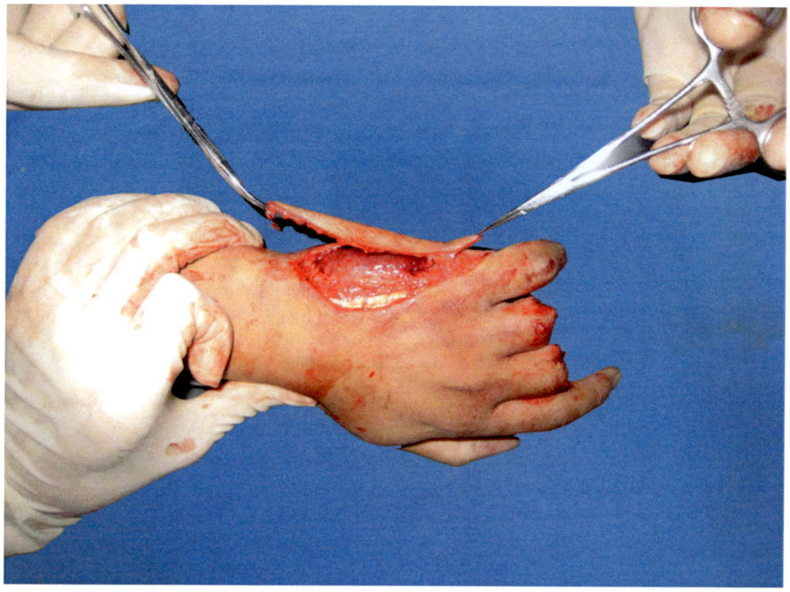

Fig. 15.7 Flap elevation

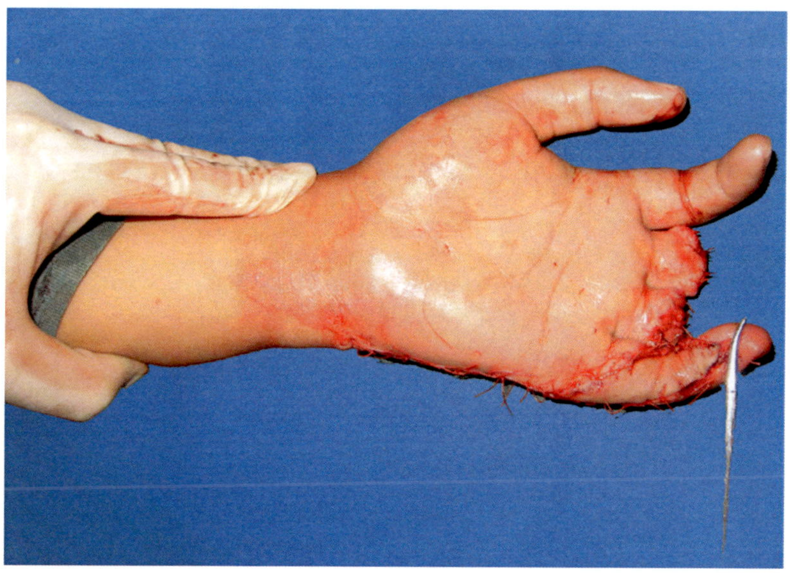

Fig. 15.8 Flap rotation

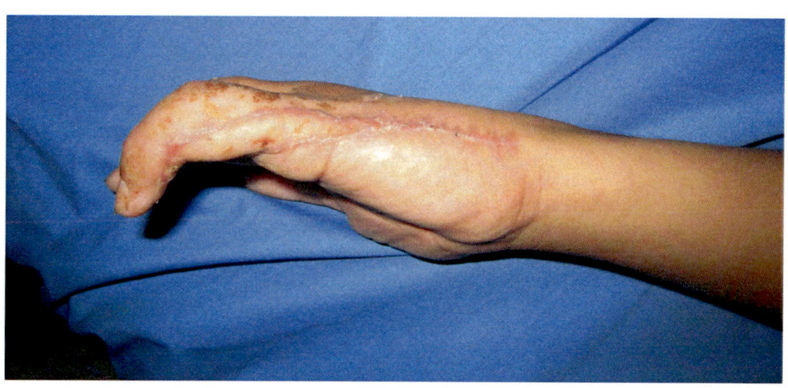

Fig. 15.9 Follow-up

Pearls

This reverse flap pedicled on the dorsal branch of the ulnar artery may be a feasible reconstructive option for loss of distal soft tissue from the ulnar digits.

Pitfalls

Raising a reversed fourth and fifth dorsal metacarpal flaps on the ulnar aspect of the hand is not always possible because of the variable arterial anatomy [5, 6]; this reverse flap pedicled by the dorsal branch of the ulnar artery may be a feasible reconstructive option for loss of distal soft tissue from the ulnar digits.

References

1. Bertelli JA, Khoury Z. Neurocutaneous island flaps in the hand: anatomical basis and preliminary results. Br J Plast Surg. 1992;45(8):586–90.
2. Murata K, Inada Y, Fukui A, Tamai S, Takakura Y. Clinical application of the reversed pedicled venous flap containing perivenous areolar tissue and/or nerve in the hand. Br J Plast Surg. 2001;54(7):615–20.
3. Okada E, Maruyama Y, Hayashi A. Stepladder dorsal metacarpal flaps for dorsal finger and hand reconstruction. Ann Plast Surg. 2002;48(1):48–52.
4. Pelissier P, Casoli V, Bakhach J, Martin D, Baudet J. Reverse dorsal digital and metacarpal flaps: a review of 27 cases. Plast Reconstr Surg. 1999;103(1):159–65.
5. Coleman SS, Anson BJ. Arterial patterns in the hand based upon a study of 650 specimens. Surg Gynecol Obstet. 1961;113:409–24.
6. Lister G. The theory of the transposition flap and its practical application in the hand. Clin Plast Surg. 1981;8(1):115–27.

16 Digital Artery Perforator Flap

As the name suggests, digital artery perforator (DAP) flaps are based off the digital arteries. The concept of DAP flaps arose from the observation that many arterial branches from the digital artery originate in the lateral aspect of the finger. These branches perforate the thin fascia and adiposal tissue, terminating in multiple arterioles in the subdermal layer [1, 2].

Koshima et al. originally reported the utility of DAP flaps for fingertip reconstruction [3].

16.1 Vascular Anatomy

The reverse adipofascial dorsal digital (RADD) flaps are nourished by dorsal communicating branches of the digital arteries, which are numerous and constant (Fig. 16.1); venous drainage depends on the parallel venous system surrounding the arterial pedicle [2, 4–14].

C. Hou et al., *Surgical Atlas of Perforator Flaps: A Microsurgical Dissection Technique*,
DOI 10.1007/978-94-017-9834-1_16, © Springer Science+Business Media Dordrecht 2015

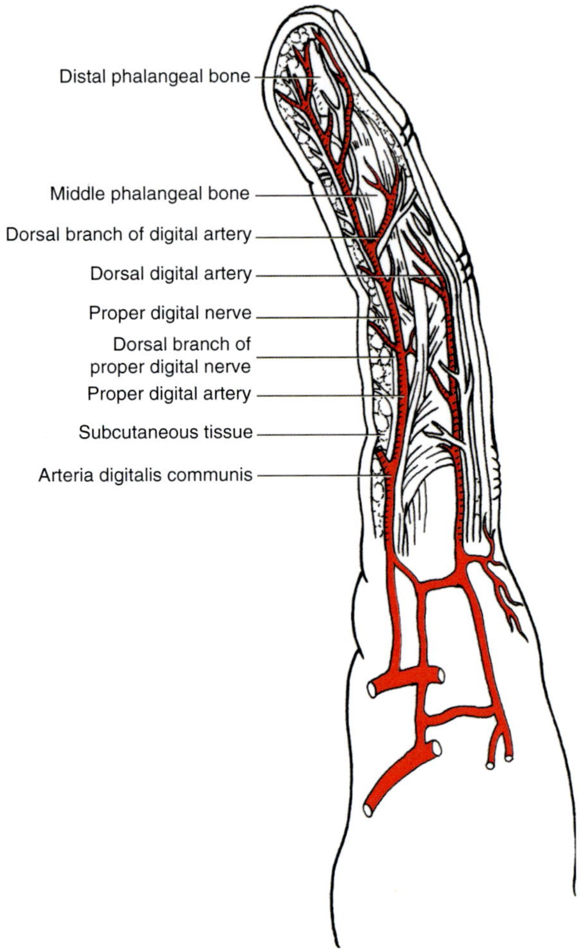

Fig. 16.1 Vascular anatomy of the digital artery

16.2 Illustrative Case

Case 1

A 39-year-old woman suffered a crush amputation of her right thumb fingertip following an accident with a metal press machine. The defect size was 3.0×2.5 cm (Fig. 16.2).

Flap Design

The flap is designed on the radial dorsal metacarpal artery perforator that located close to the defect (Fig. 16.3). The selected perforator is marked at the level of the metacarpal neck (Fig. 16.4).

Flap Elevation

The flap is elevated from proximal to distal under tourniquet control in the loose areolar tissue plane superficial to the extensor tendon paratenon (Fig. 16.5). Large veins at the edge of the flap are avoided because these veins only add to stasis within the flap (Fig. 16.6).

Flap Transfer and Insetting

The flap is then rotated into the defect and anchored loosely to the edges of the defect with the interphalangeal and metacarpophalangeal joints in extension (Fig. 16.7).

Follow-Up

The flap survived smoothly (Fig. 16.8).

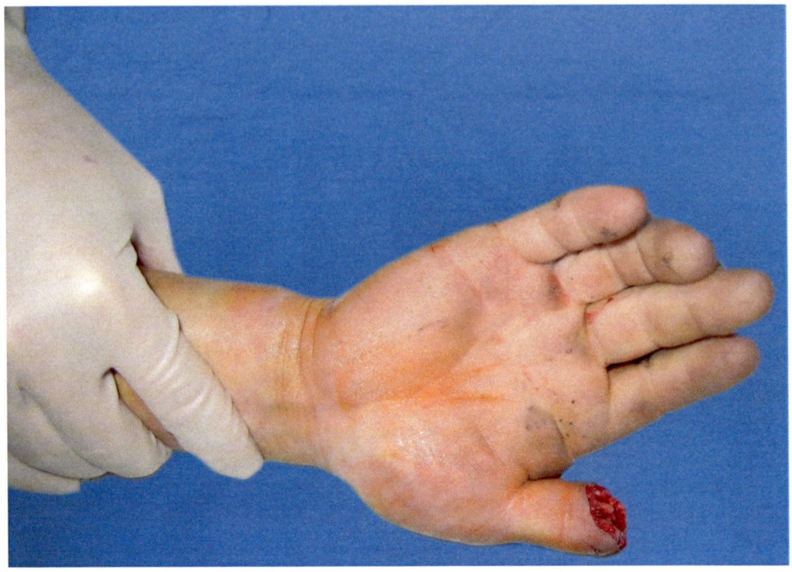

Fig. 16.2 Preoperative view

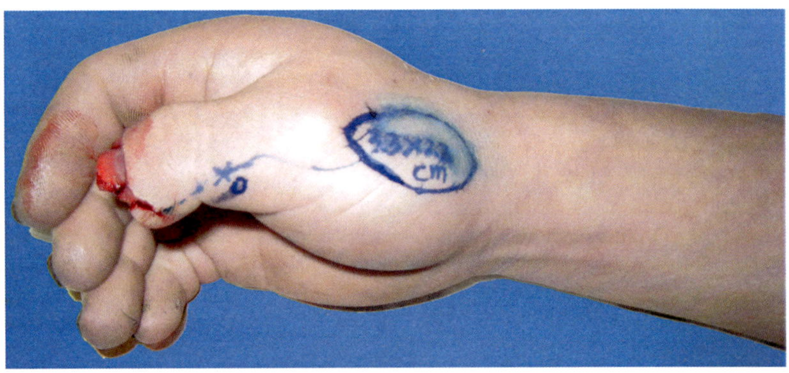

Fig. 16.3 Flap design

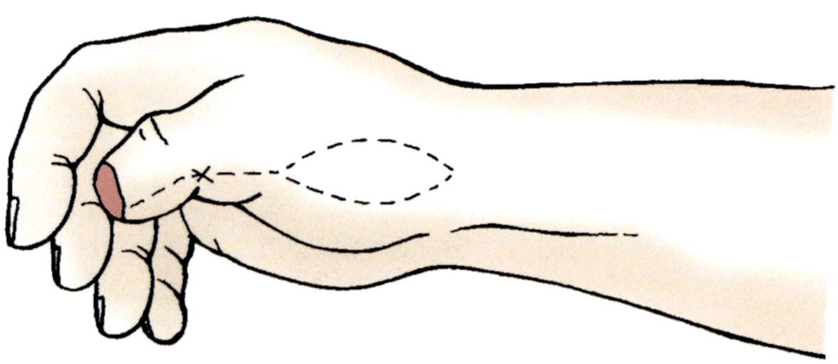

Fig. 16.4 Schematic drawing of the flap design

Fig. 16.5 Flap elevation

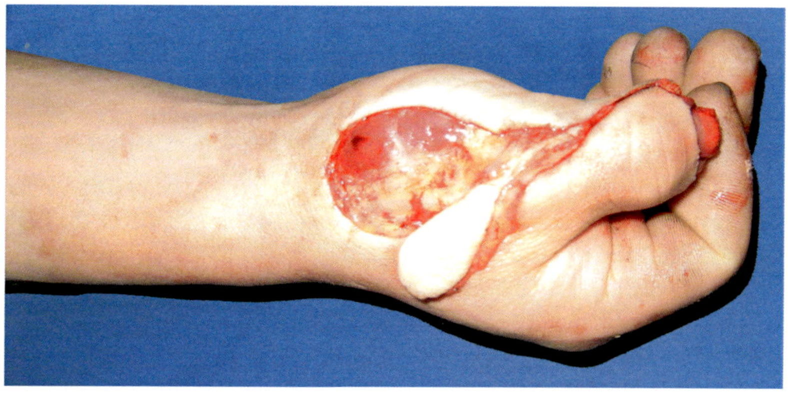

Fig. 16.6 Schematic drawing of the flap elevation

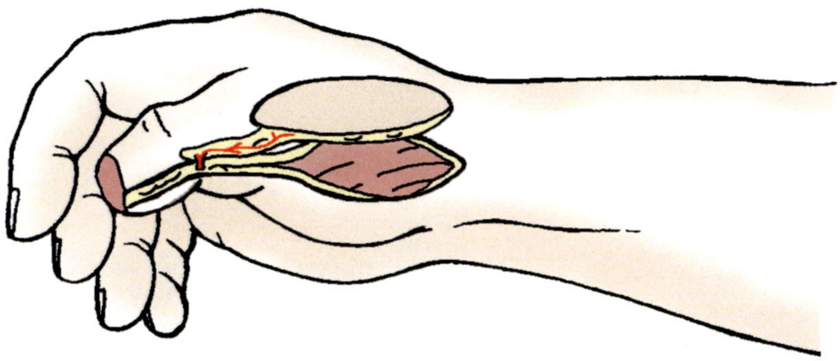

Fig. 16.7 Flap rotation

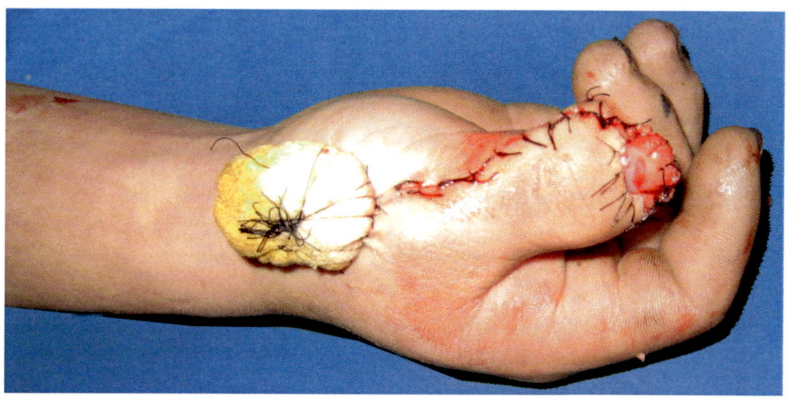

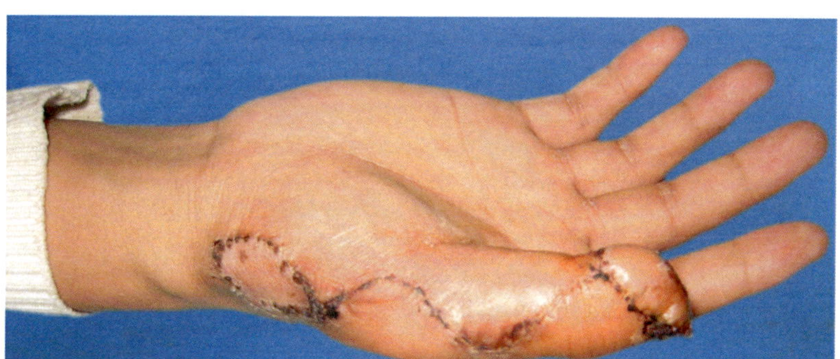

Fig. 16.8 Follow-up

Case 2

A 27-year-old man suffered crush injury of the dorsum of his left thumb (Fig. 16.9).

The defect size was 3.0 × 2.0 cm.

Flap Design

A distally based flap was designed (Fig. 16.10). The pedicle was based just medial and proximal to the defect (Fig. 16.11).

Flap Elevation

The designed flap is elevated superficial to the digital neurovascular bundle (Fig. 16.12). At the side of the flap most proximal to the defect, the DAP closest to the defect is preserved as the pedicle vessel. Because the pedicle was very narrow in diameter, it was necessary to include periareolar soft tissue at the base of the pedicle (Fig. 16.13).

Flap Transfer

The perforator-based island flap is then rotated 90° to cover the defect (Fig. 16.14).

Flap Insetting

The donor site is closed with split-thickness skin graft (Fig. 16.15).

Follow-Up

The flap survived smoothly (Fig. 16.16).

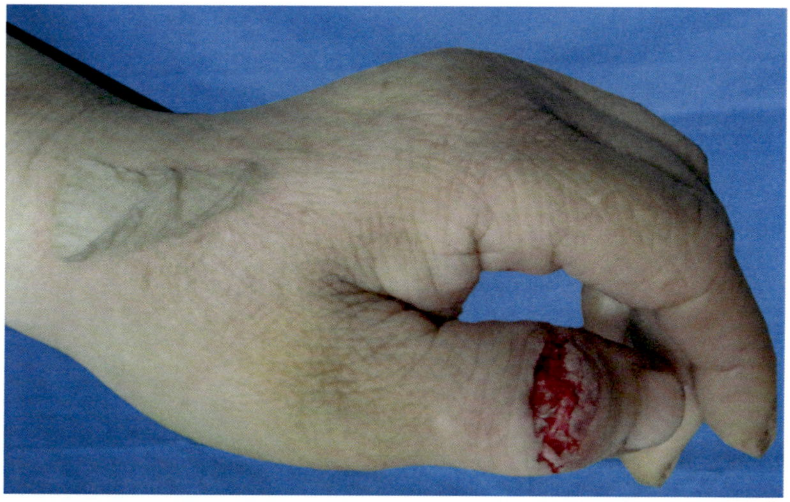

Fig. 16.9 Preoperative view

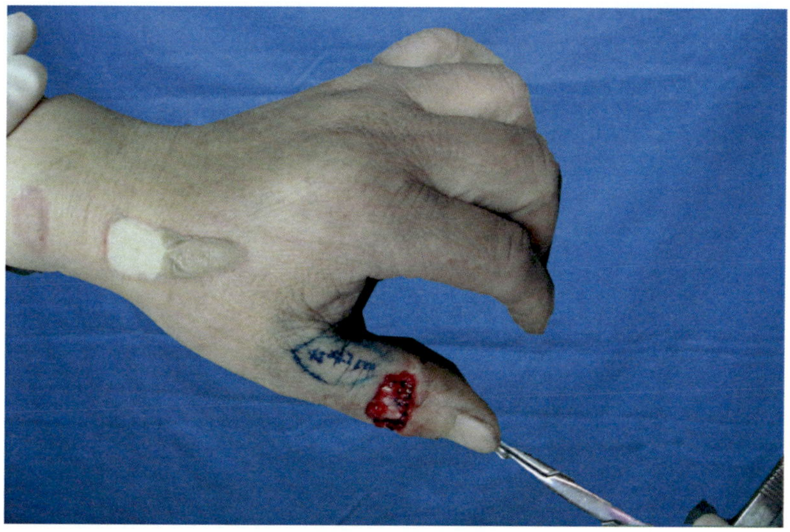

Fig. 16.10 Flap design

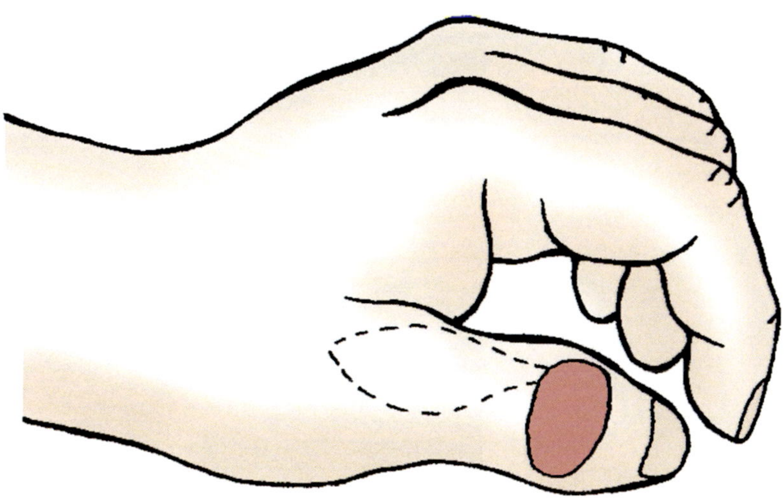

Fig. 16.11 Schematic drawing of the flap design

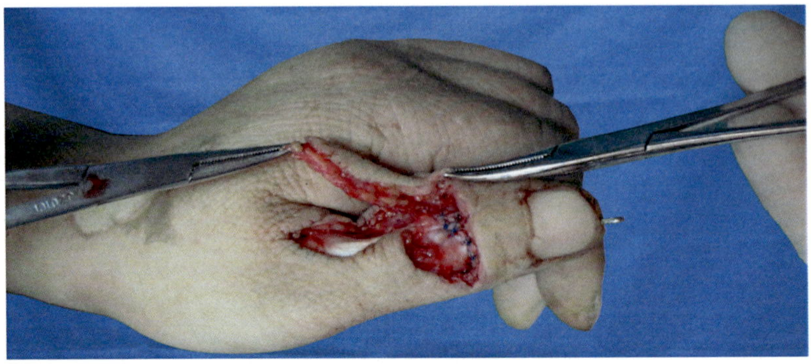

Fig. 16.12 Flap elevation

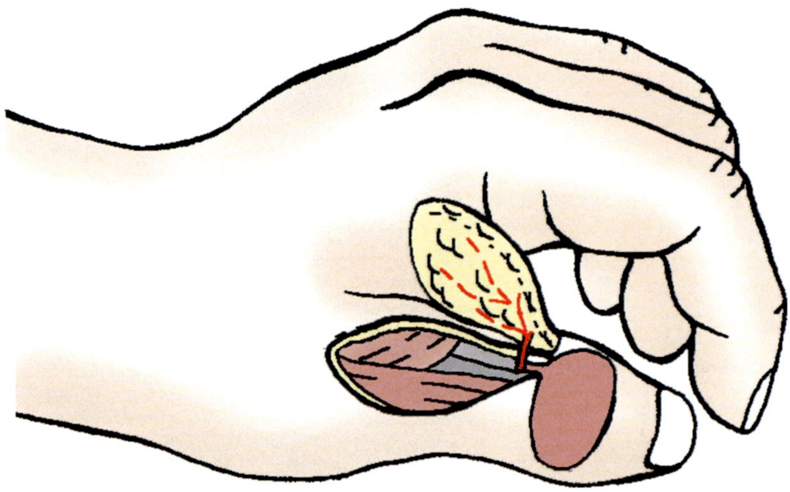

Fig. 16.13 Schematic drawing of the flap elevation

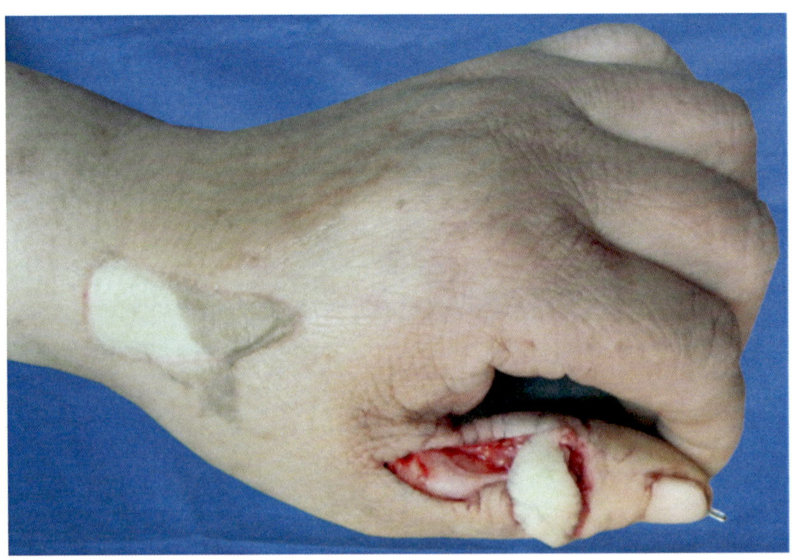

Fig. 16.14 Flap rotation

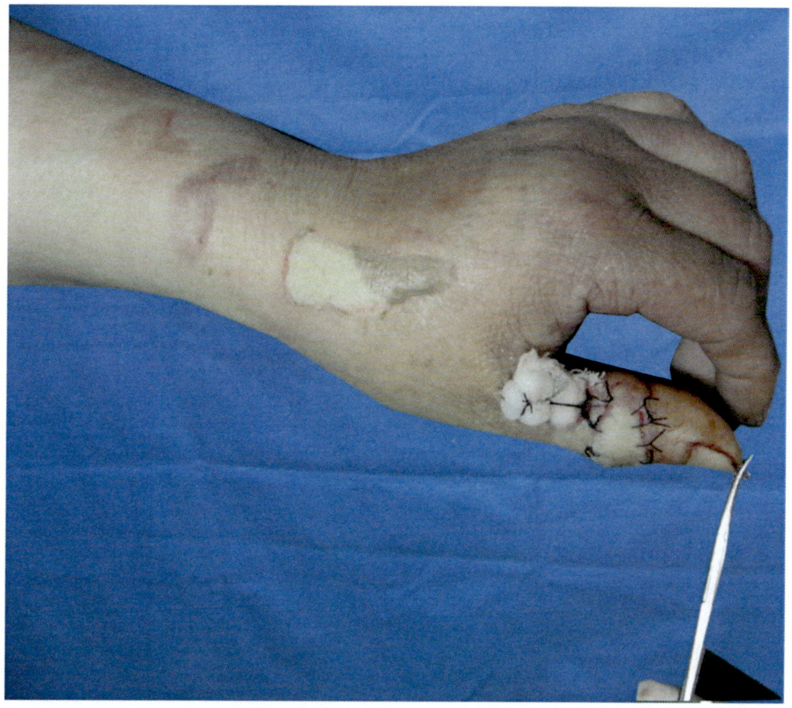

Fig. 16.15 Postoperative view

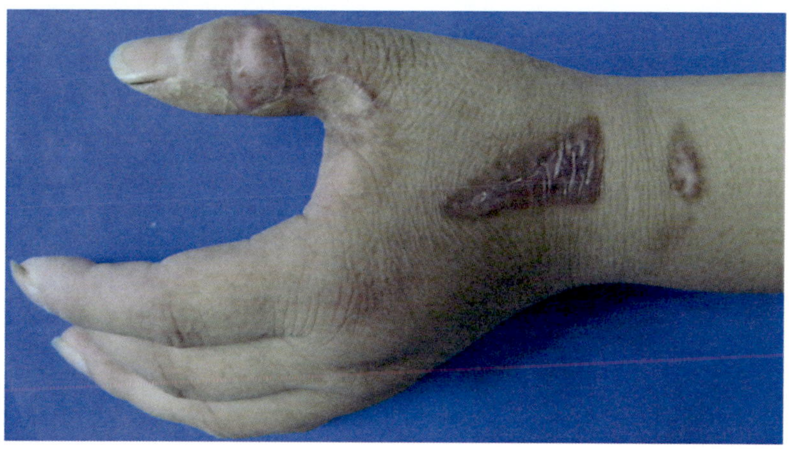

Fig. 16.16 Follow-up

Case 3

A 30-year-old man suffered crush amputations of his right middle and index fingers following an accident with a book press machine.

The fingertip of the middle finger was amputated; the remaining stump had a palmar skin and soft tissue defect. The index finger was amputated proximal to the level of the distal interphalangeal (DIP) joint. Due to the severe extent of the crush injury, fingertip replantation could not be performed for either finger. We therefore elected to attempt finger reconstruction using DAP flaps (Fig. 16.17).

Flap Design

DAP flap reconstruction was performed to maintain finger length (Fig. 16.18). A 2.0 × 1.6 cm DAP flap was designed on the ulnar side of both proximal phalanx (Fig. 16.19).

Flap Elevation (Fig. 16.20)

The designed flap is elevated superficial to the digital neurovascular bundle (Fig. 16.21).

Flap Transfer

The flaps were rotated 180° to cover the defects (Fig. 16.22) without further bone shortening (Fig. 16.23).

The flap survived smoothly (Fig. 16.24).

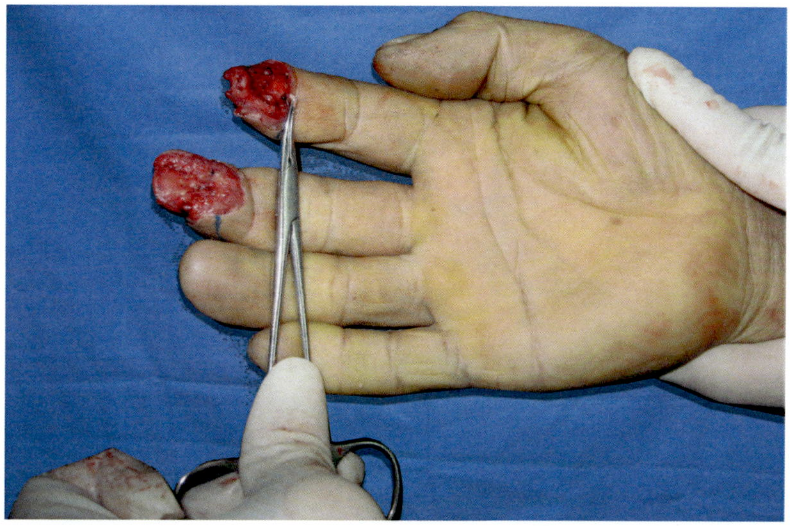

Fig. 16.17 Preoperative view

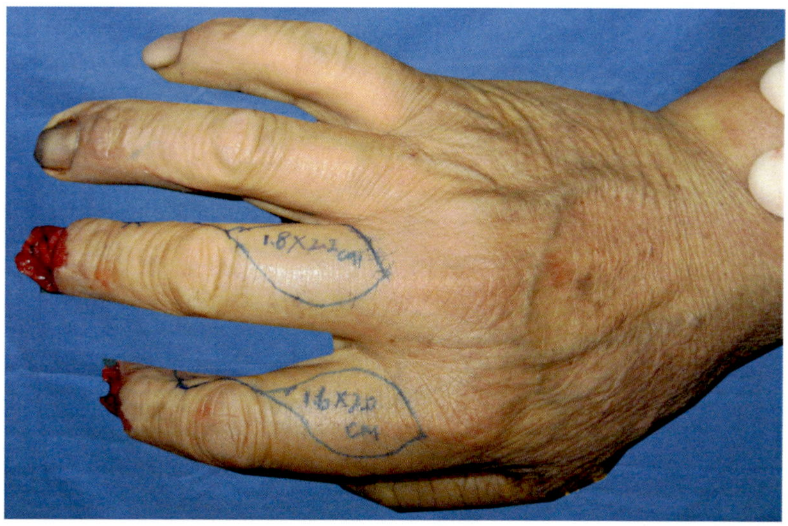

Fig. 16.18 Flap design

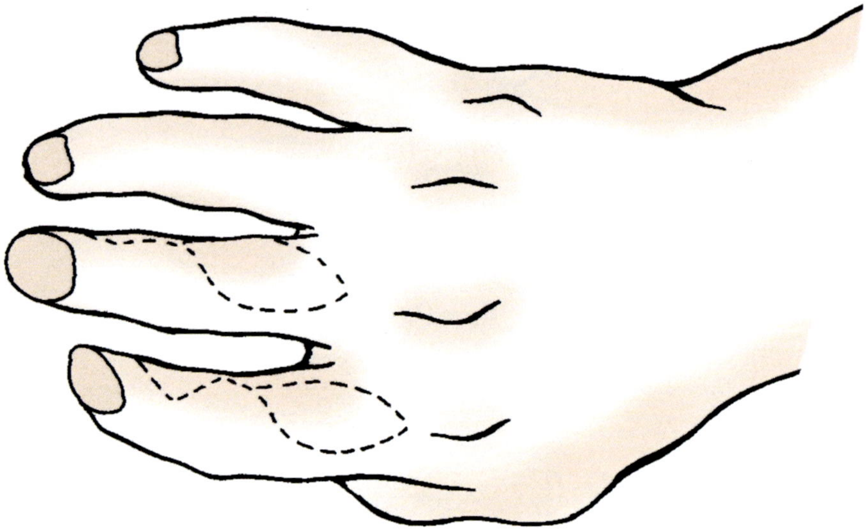

Fig. 16.19 Schematic drawing of the flap design

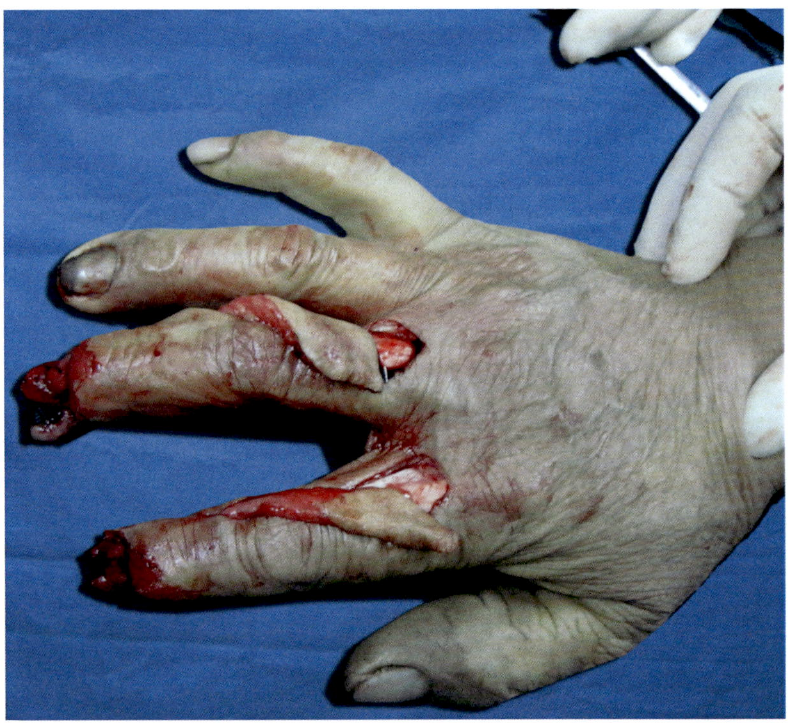

Fig. 16.20 Flap elevation

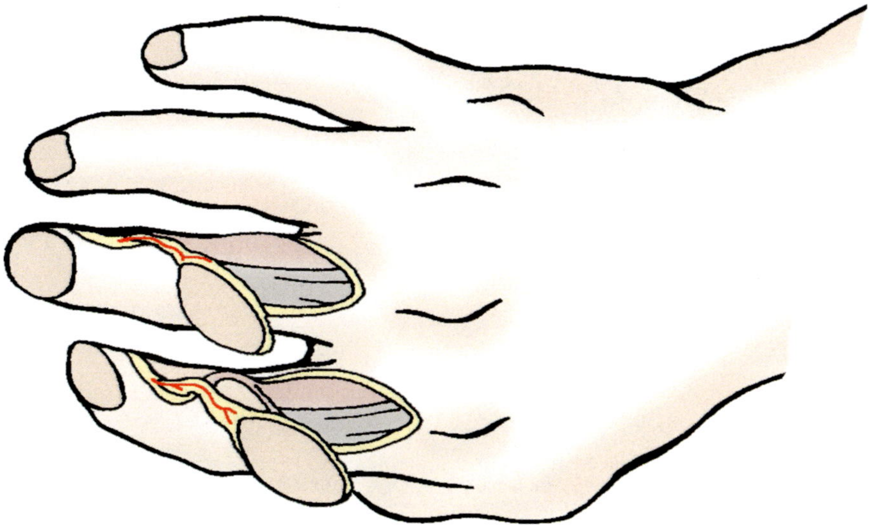

Fig. 16.21 Schematic drawing of the flap elevation

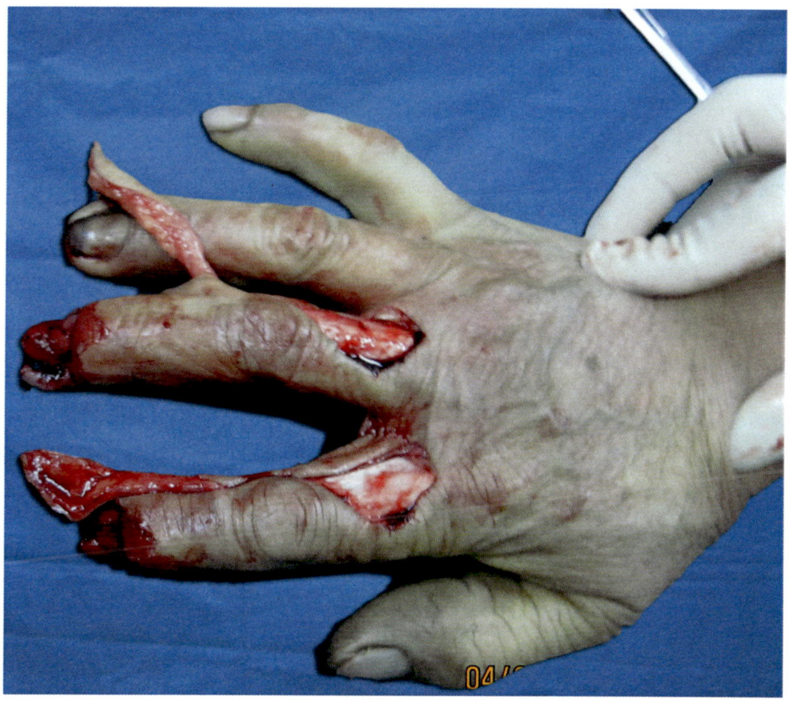

Fig. 16.22 Flaps transfer

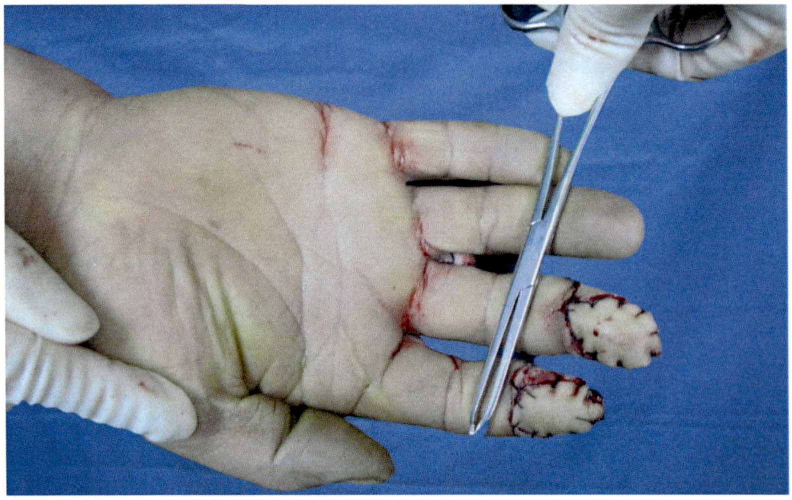

Fig. 16.23 Flap insetting

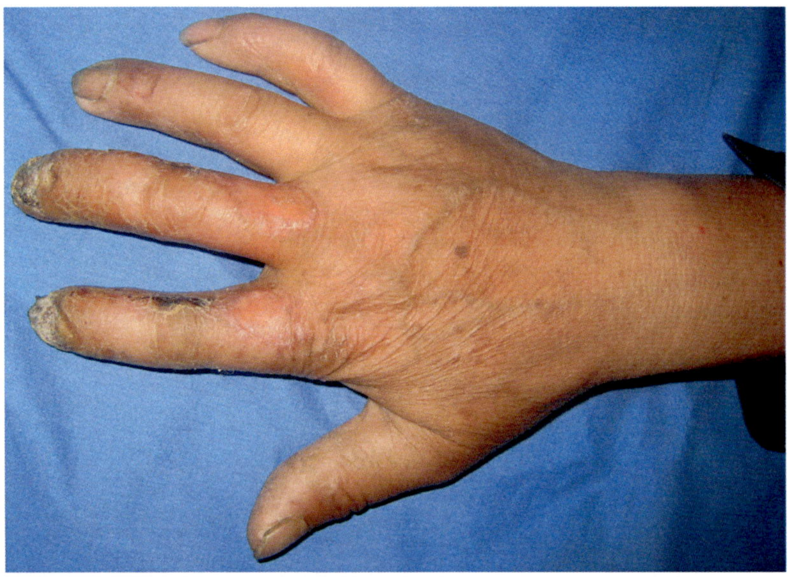

Fig. 16.24 Follow-up

Case 4

A 27-year-old man suffered crush amputations of his left middle and little fingers.

The fingertip of the middle finger was amputated, and the remaining stump had a palmar skin and soft tissue defect. The little finger was amputated proximal to the level of the distal interphalangeal (DIP) joint (Fig. 16.25).

Flap Design

A 2×1.5 cm DAP flap was designed on the ulnar side of the ring finger stump (Fig. 16.26). A 1.5×1.5 cm DAP flap was designed on the ulnar side of the little finger stump (Fig. 16.27).

Flap Elevation (Fig. 16.28)

The designed flap is elevated superficial to the digital neurovascular bundle (Fig. 16.29).

Flap Transfer and Insetting

The perforator-based island flaps were rotated 180° (Fig. 16.30) to cover the defect (Fig. 16.31).

Follow-Up

The flap survived smoothly (Fig. 16.32).

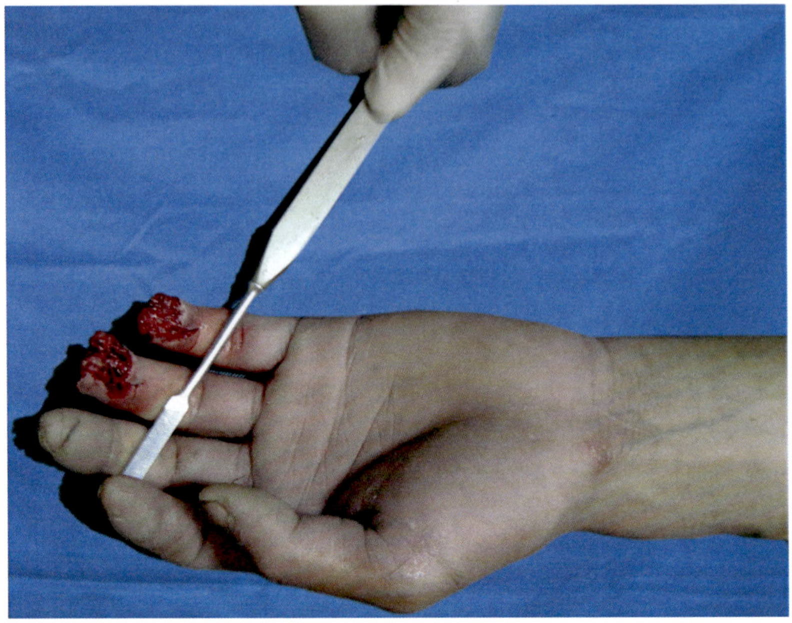

Fig. 16.25 Preoperative view

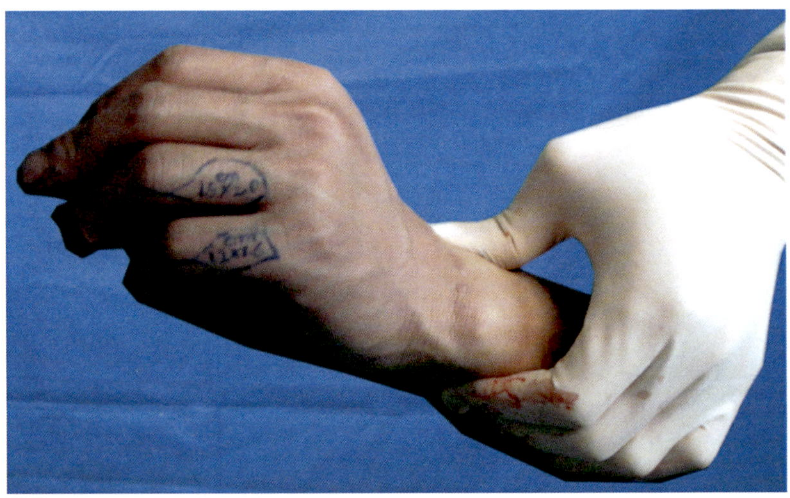

Fig. 16.26 Flap design

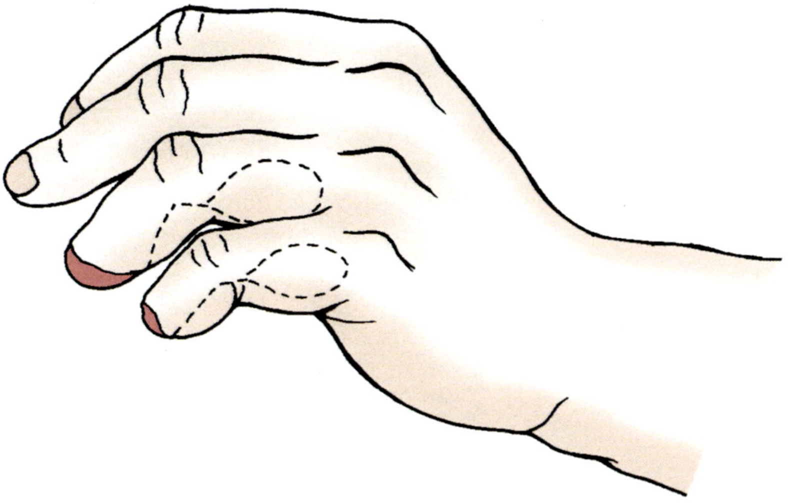

Fig. 16.27 Schematic drawing of the flap design

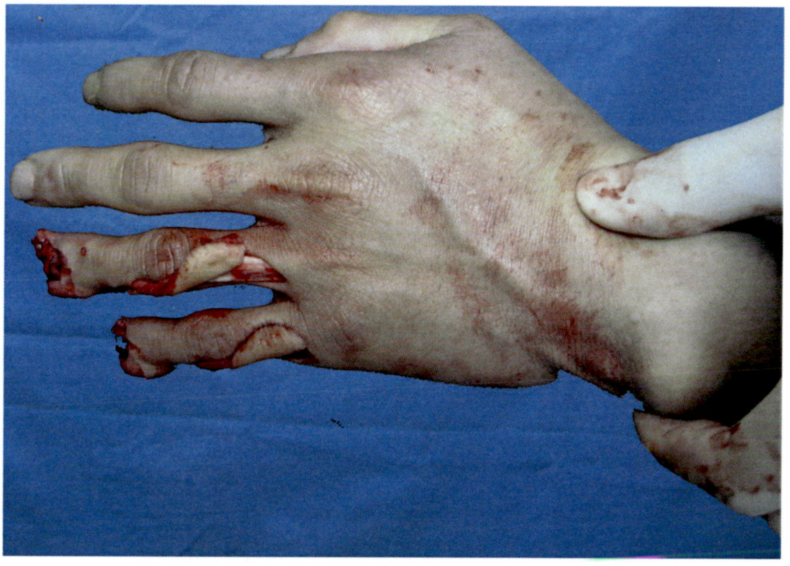

Fig. 16.28 Flap elevation

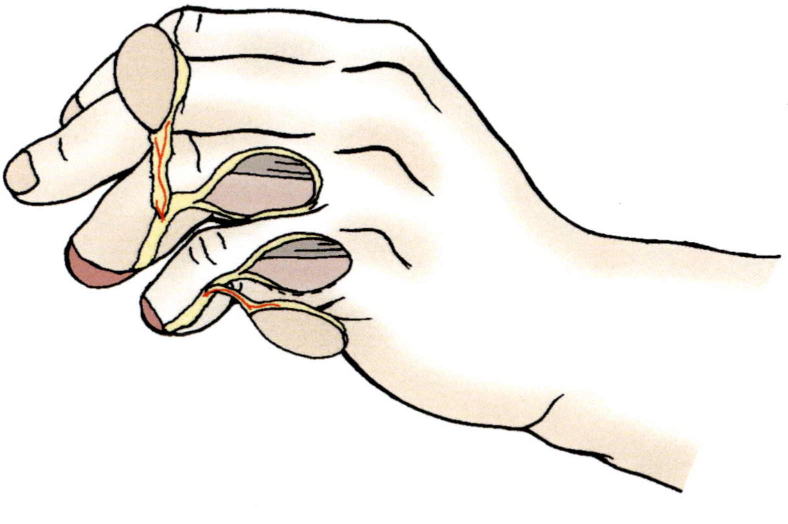

Fig. 16.29 Schematic drawing of the flap elevation

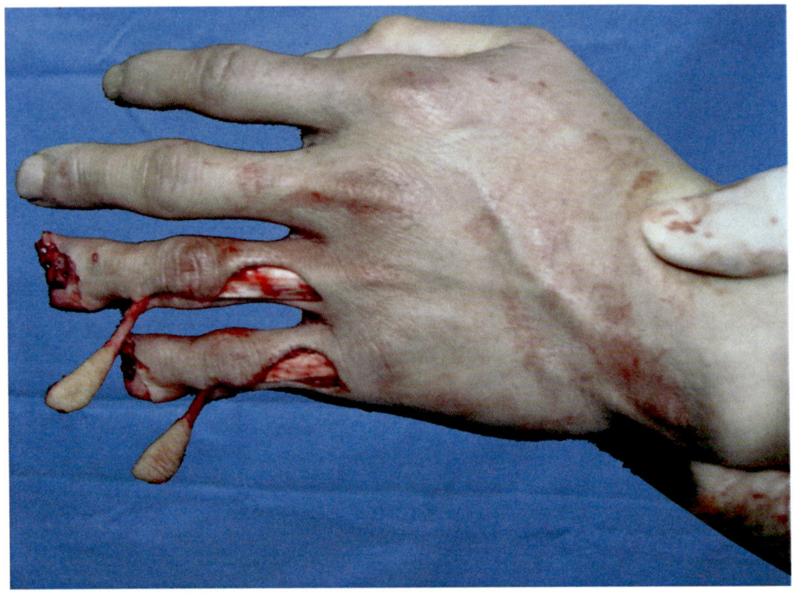

Fig. 16.30 Flap transfer

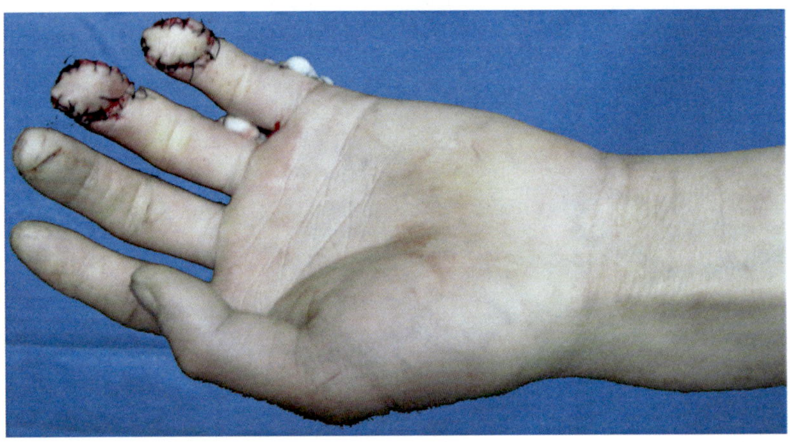

Fig. 16.31 Flap insetting

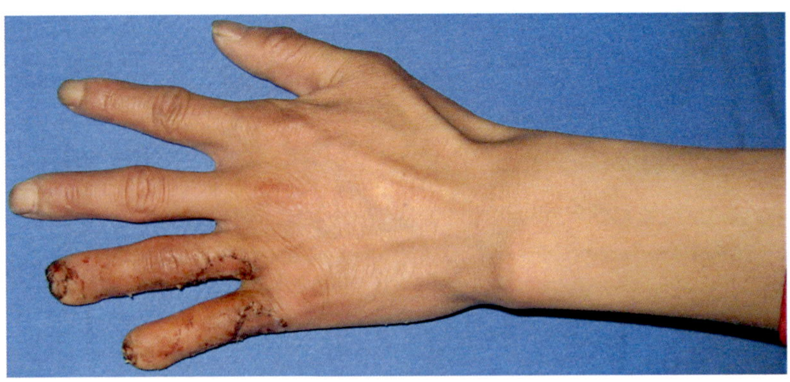

Fig. 16.32 Follow-up

> **Pearls**
> The RADD flaps were used for the defects over proximal interphalangeal joint or interphalangeal joint at the thumb and further distally [15–18].

> **Pitfalls**
> It is important to ensure that there is no injury (e.g., contusion to the dorsal skin, previous injection of a local anesthetic, deep laceration extending into the webspace, or metacarpal neck or head fracture) in the vicinity of the selected perforator [19, 20].
>
> Meticulous hemostasis must be secured [20–25].
>
> Minimize any compression of the flap or the bridge segment [5, 26].

References

1. Endo T, Kojima T, Hirase Y. Vascular anatomy of the finger dorsum and a new idea for coverage of the finger pulp defect that restores sensation. J Hand Surg. 1992;17(5):927–32.
2. Strauch B, de Moura W. Arterial system of the fingers. J Hand Surg. 1990;15(1):148–54.
3. Koshima I, Urushibara K, Fukuda N, et al. Digital artery perforator flaps for fingertip reconstructions. Plast Reconstr Surg. 2006;118(7):1579–84.
4. Ozdemir R, Kilinc H, Sensoz O, Unlu RE, Baran CN. Innervated dorsal adipofascial turnover flap for fingertip amputations. Ann Plast Surg. 2001;46(1):9–14.
5. Chen C, Tang P, Zhao G. Direct and reversed dorsal digital island flaps: a review of 65 cases. Injury. 2014;45(12):2013–7.
6. Lu YJ, Hong GX, Xu NW, Hu ZY, Shao L. Reconstruction of finger pulp defect with reversed fasciocutaneous island flap from same finger. Chinese journal of traumatology = Zhonghua chuang shang za zhi/Chin Med Assoc. 2007;10(2):82–5.
7. Hu H, Zhang D. [Classification of finger flaps and its use in emergency treatment for finger injuries]. Zhongguo xiu fu chong jian wai ke za zhi = Zhongguo xiufu chongjian waike zazhi = Chin J Reparative Reconstr Surg. 2006;20(12):1196–8.
8. Hu HT. [Emergency repair of finger soft tissue loss with island flaps]. Chinese journal of plastic surgery Zhonghua zheng xing wai ke za zhi = Zhonghua zhengxing waike zazhi = Chin J Plast Surg. 2004;20(6):431–3.
9. Casoli V, Verolino P, Pelissier P, et al. The retrograde neurocutaneous island flap of the dorsal branch of the ulnar nerve: anatomical basis and clinical application. Surg Radiol Anat SRA. 2004;26(1):8–13.
10. Du Y, Feng X, Xu G. [Clinical application of the reversed digital arterial island flap with digital vein and digital dorsal nerve anastomosis]. Zhonghua zheng xing wai ke za zhi = Zhonghua zhengxing waike zazhi = Chin J Plast Surg. 2001;17(5):267–8.
11. Yang D, Morris SF. Reversed dorsal digital and metacarpal island flaps supplied by the dorsal cutaneous branches of the palmar digital artery. Ann Plast Surg. 2001;46(4):444–9.
12. Brunelli F, Vigasio A, Valenti P, Brunelli GR. Arterial anatomy and clinical application of the dorsoulnar flap of the thumb. J Hand Surg. 1999;24(4):803–11.
13. Zhu L, Xu Q, Kou W, Ning B, Jia T. Outcome of free digital artery perforator flap transfer for reconstruction of fingertip defects. Indian J Orthop. 2014;48(6):594–8.
14. Lee SH, Jang JH, Kim JI, Cheon SJ. Modified anterograde pedicle advancement flap in fingertip injury. J Hand Surg Eur Vo. 2014;25(2):347–51.
15. Vuppalapati G, Oberlin C, Balakrishnan G. "Distally based dorsal hand flaps": clinical experience, cadaveric studies and an update. Br J Plast Surg. 2004;57(7):653–67.
16. Zhang Y, Xin CT. [Digital artery bilobed flap for the treatment of skin degloving injury of thumb]. Zhongguo gu shang = Chin J Orthop Traumatol. 2014;27(4):307–10.
17. Shen H, Shen Z, Wang Y, Zhang K, Zhang Z, Dai X. Extended reverse dorsal metacarpal artery flap for coverage of finger defects distal to the proximal interphalangeal joint. Ann Plast Surg. 2014;72(5):529–36.
18. Jiang Q, Feng M, Jiang Z, Liu J. [Repairing degloving injury of distal phalanx with homodigital bilobed flaps tiled]. Zhongguo xiu fu chong jian wai ke za zhi = Zhongguo xiufu chongjian waike zazhi = Chin J Reparative Reconstr Surg. 2012;26(7):806–9.
19. Chen C, Tang P, Zhang X. The dorsal homodigital island flap based on the dorsal branch of the digital artery: a review of 166 cases. Plast Reconstr Surg. 2014;133(4):519e–29.
20. Feng SM, Gu JX, Liu HJ, et al. Treatment of distal fingertip degloving injuries using a cross-finger flap based on the dorsal branch of the proper digital artery at the middle phalanx. J Reconstr Microsurg. 2013;29(9):623–30.
21. Zheng DW, Li ZC, Sun F, Shi RJ, Shou KS. Use of a distal ulnar artery perforator-based bilobed free flap for repairing complex digital defects. J Hand Surg. 2014;39(11):2235–42.

22. Chen C, Zhang W, Tang P. Direct and reversed dorsal digito-metacarpal flaps: a review of 24 cases. Injury. 2014;45(4):805–12.
23. Chen C, Tang P, Zhang L. Reconstruction of a soft tissue defect in the finger using the heterodigital neurocutaneous island flap. Injury. 2013;44(11):1607–14.
24. Chen C, Tang P, Zhang L. Use of a bipedicled nerve flap taken from the dorsum of the digit for reconstruction of neurocutaneous defect in the adjacent finger. J Plast Reconstr Aesthet Surg JPRAS. 2013;66(10):1322–9.
25. Chen C, Tang P, Zhang L, Li X, Zheng Y. Repair of multiple finger defects using the dorsal homodigital island flaps. Injury. 2013;44(11):1582–8.
26. Liu Y, Jiao H, Ji X, et al. A comparative study of four types of free flaps from the ipsilateral extremity for finger reconstruction. PLoS One. 2014;9(8):e104014.

17 Perforator Flaps in the Lateral Thoracic Region

Cutaneous branches from the thoracodorsal and lateral thoracic arteries were first mentioned by de Coninck et al., and the flaps based on these arteries have been known as thoracodorsal skin flaps, thoracodorsal axillary flaps, and lateral thoracic flaps [1–5].

17.1 Vascular Anatomy

The subscapular artery arises from the axillary artery and divides into the thoracodorsal and the circumflex scapular arteries (Fig. 17.1). The thoracodorsal artery penetrates the latissimus dorsi muscle about 8–14 cm from the bifurcation of the subscapular artery into the circumflex scapular and thoracodorsal. Shortly before it enters the muscle, the vascular bundles send a branch to the serratus anterior muscle. The latissimus dorsi muscle is nourished by two main muscular branches from the thoracodorsal artery: a lateral branch running parallel to the anterior border and a horizontal branch passing obliquely to the dorsal and medial part of the muscle. They give multiple terminals to the skin as perforators through the muscle along the course of branches, and these musculocutaneous perforators are located at intervals in the back area. Septocutaneous perforators arise from the branch to the serratus anterior or other cutaneous branches, and they reach the skin between the latissimus dorsi and serratus anterior muscles.

Cutaneous branches originate from the main thoracodorsal artery or from the branch to the serratus anterior.

They also supply septocutaneous perforators or direct cutaneous perforators.

C. Hou et al., *Surgical Atlas of Perforator Flaps: A Microsurgical Dissection Technique*,
DOI 10.1007/978-94-017-9834-1_17, © Springer Science+Business Media Dordrecht 2015

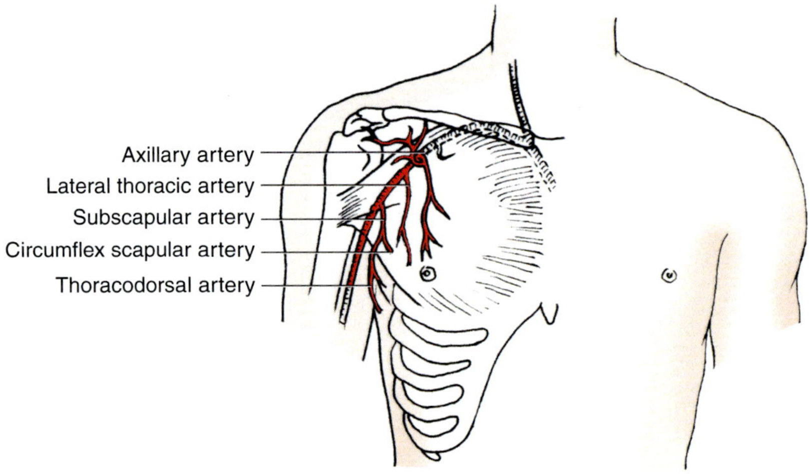

Fig. 17.1 Vascular anatomy of the thoracodorsal and lateral thoracic artery

17.2 Illustrative Case

A 30-year-old male presents with complete left upper extremity amputation at proximal humerus after industrial grinder accident. The patient was placed in a lateral decubitus position with the ipsilateral upper extremity positioned freely and exposing the axilla by using adequate supports and padding, taking great care to avoid compression of the axillary neurovascular structures. The anterior border of the latissimus dorsi muscle and the center of the axillary fossa are marked (Fig. 17.2).

The expected area is 8–10 cm from the center of the axillary fossa and within 2 cm posterior to the anterior border of the muscle (Fig. 17.3).

Flap Elevation

An incision is made along the anterior border of the designed flap and the subcutaneous layer is split gently to the level of the fascia overlying the muscle.

Vertical dissection is carried to the plane of deep fascia using a sharp instrument until a pulsating perforator is detected. Great care is required near the expected area of the perforator. The dissection continues in the same plane with vertical traction of the skin until a reliable perforator is found. Tiny vascular tributaries and the collateral nerve branch can be good indicators for reaching the reliable perforator, and the nerve can be preserved for a sensate flap (Fig. 17.4). After the identification of the reliable musculocutaneous perforator, it is traced distally to isolate the point of entry into the fat and skin (Fig. 17.5).

Flap Transfer

The dissection of the pedicle proceeds through the muscle. Muscle fascicles are spread gently following the course of the dissection and tiny muscular branches are carefully tied or cauterized with a bipolar instrument at a safe distance. Initial transmuscular dissection requires great care until the diameter of the perforator increases underneath several muscular fascicles. The thoracodorsal nerve is separated from the vascular pedicle and dissection proceeds proximally by retracting the muscle and adipose tissue in the axilla until the length and the diameter match those of the recipient vessels (Fig. 17.6).

Flap Insetting

The flap rotated 180° to cover the defect. The donor site was closed directly (Fig. 17.7).

Follow-Up

The flap survived eventually (Fig. 17.8).

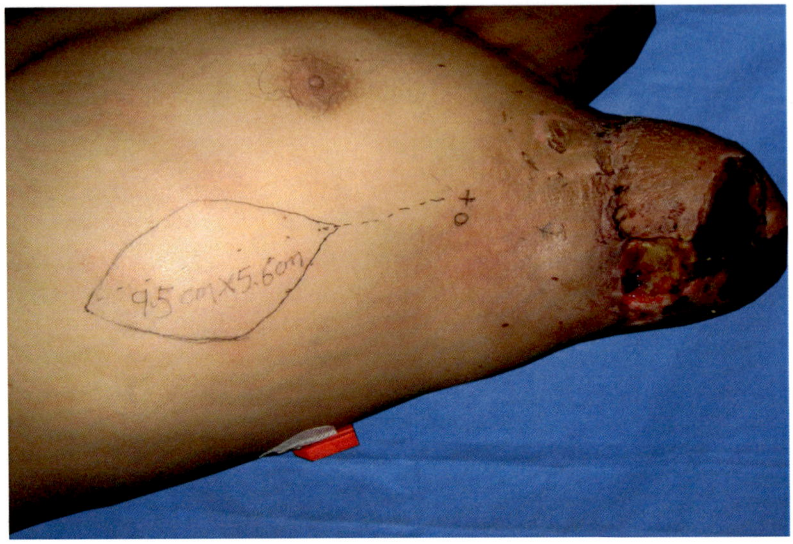

Fig. 17.2 Flap design

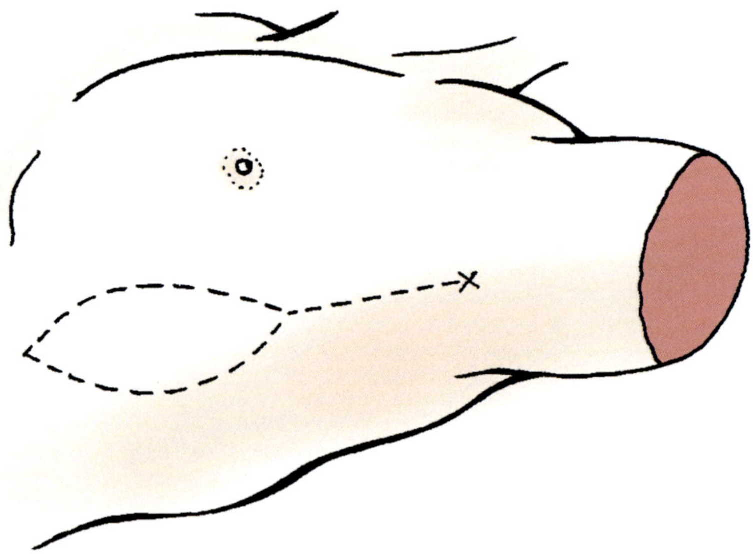

Fig. 17.3 Schematic drawing of the flap design

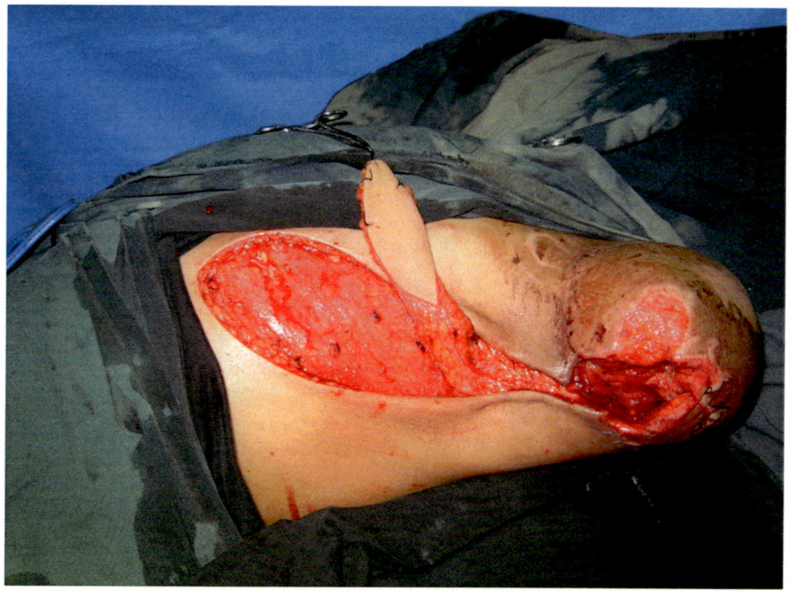

Fig. 17.4 Flap elevation

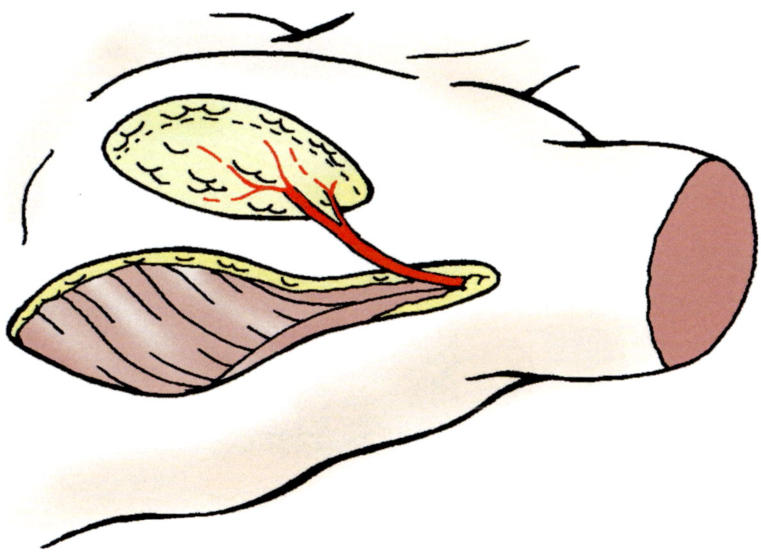

Fig. 17.5 Schematic drawing of the flap elevation

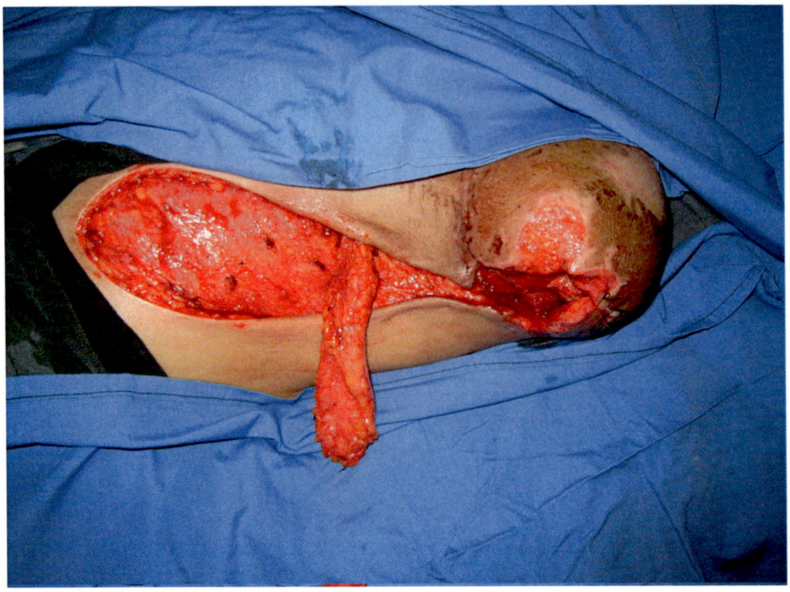

Fig. 17.6 Flap transfer

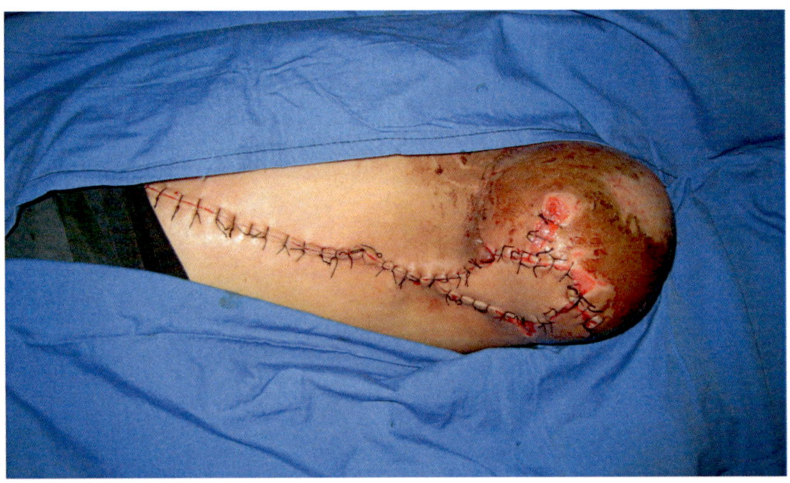

Fig. 17.7 Flap rotation

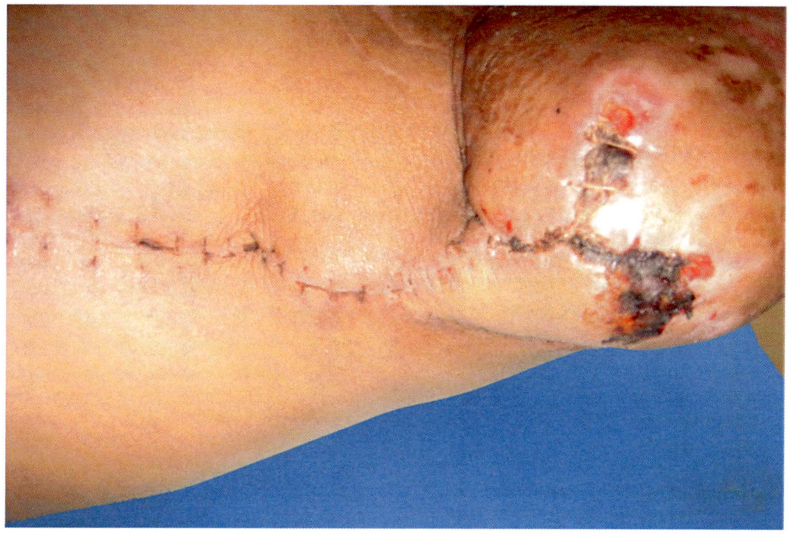

Fig. 17.8 Follow-up

Pearls

It enabled controlled resurfacing with a thin flap.

Various patterns and compositions can be harvested and used to reconstruct defects requiring different tissue arrangements and tissue types.

Sensate flap can be harvested.

Long pedicle can be obtained through transmuscular perforator pedicle dissection.

Perforator dissection allows for preservation of muscle and motor nerves and minimizes donor-site morbidity. The donor site can be closed primarily up to 10 cm, resulting in an acceptable linear scar and no functional deficits.

Pitfalls

It is helpful if the surgeon can distinguish an intercostal from a reliable or usable perforator early on to avoid wasting time. Intercostal perforators are less in number and not so distinct as reliable perforators from the thoracodorsal vascular system. The intercostal perforator exit is located anterior to the septocutaneous perforator row. Even though it looks definite, in most cases it is not an intercostal perforator but a septocutaneous perforator.

As the pulsation of the reliable perforator can easily disappear with a spasm, the perforator pedicle should be frequently irrigated with a vasodilator solution. In spite of this, the pedicle is quite sensitive to spasm or congestion. Initial temporary ischemia may turn to a mild congestion and may remain for several days or more.

References

1. Bhattacharya S, Bhagia SP, Bhatnagar SK, Chandra R. The lateral thoracic region flap. Br J Plast Surg. 1990;43(2):162–8.
2. de Coninck A, Boeckx W. Autotransplants using vascular microsutures. Acta Chir Belg. 1975;74(6):581–6.
3. Harii K, Torii S, Sekiguchi J. The free lateral thoracic flap. Plast Reconstr Surg. 1978;62(2):212–22.
4. Maxwell GP, Stueber K, Hoopes JE. A free latissimus dorsi myocutaneous flap: case report. Plast Reconstr Surg. 1978;62(3):462–6.
5. Taylor GI, Daniel RK. The anatomy of several free flap donor sites. Plast Reconstr Surg. 1975;56(3):243–53.

Deep Inferior Epigastric Artery Perforator (DIEP) Flap

18

Since the deep inferior epigastric artery perforator (DIEP) flap was first described in 1989 by Koshima et al. [1], the DIEP flap preserves abdominal wall function without sacrificing the functional muscles, has been proved to be a reliable option for reconstructive field, and becomes very popular in breast, head, and neck, as well as vaginal reconstruction in the field of plastic surgery [2–9].

Indications of this perforator flap with a short pedicle were superficial skin defects of the lower extremities, scalp, abdomen, or head and neck [10–13].

18.1 Vascular Anatomy

The deep inferior epigastric artery (DIEA) branches off from the external iliac artery opposite the deep circumflex iliac artery (DCIA). After crossing behind the lateral border, it enters the rectus sheath by passing anterior to the arcuate line midway between the pubis and the umbilicus. Generally, the deep inferior epigastric artery divides into two large branches (sometimes three), below the level of the umbilicus, that give off perforating vessels to the skin and muscle branches. The largest perforators (with diameters of 0.6 mm) are located within 6 cm of the umbilicus, in the medial one-third of the rectus muscle. The original free paraumbilical perforator flap described by Koshima et al. was based on a single paraumbilical perforator vessel that exhibits a suprafascial course after emerging from the anterior rectus fascia (Fig. 18.1).

C. Hou et al., *Surgical Atlas of Perforator Flaps: A Microsurgical Dissection Technique*,
DOI 10.1007/978-94-017-9834-1_18, © Springer Science+Business Media Dordrecht 2015

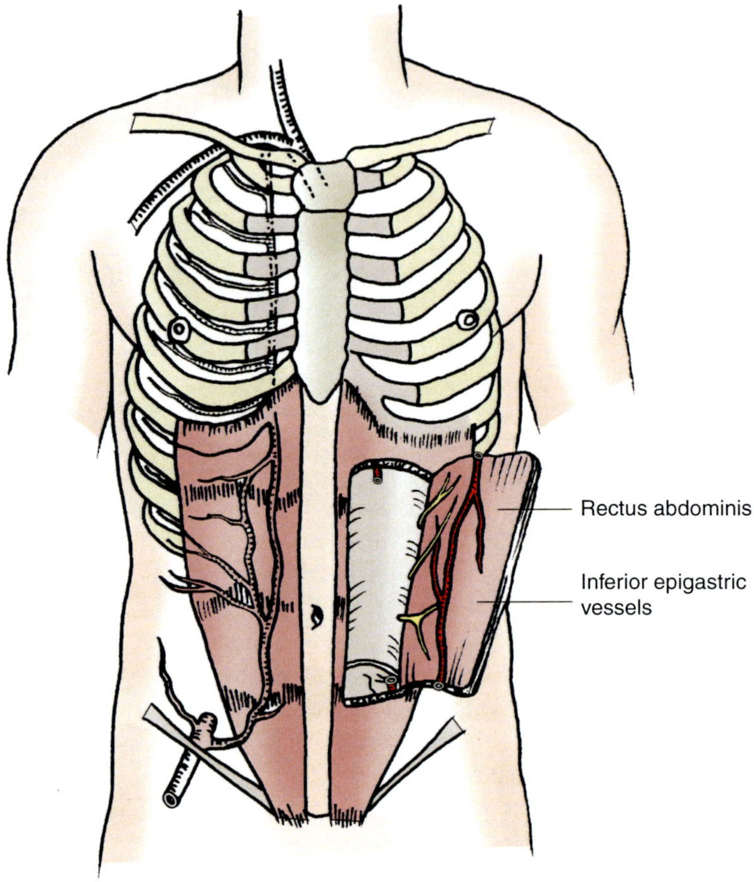

Fig. 18.1 Vascular anatomy of the deep inferior epigastric artery

18.2 Illustrative Case

An 8-year-old boy was a victim of a motorcycle accident, which resulted in a skin defect on the dorsum of his right foot, exposing the metatarsal bones, and a defect of the extensor tendons. The wound was first managed with surgical debridement and VSD. Reconstructive surgery was performed 7 days after the injury (Fig. 18.2).

Flap Design

After thorough debridement of the necrotic tissue, the extensor tendons were fixed and the skin defect was treated with a 15×9 cm oblique DIEP flap which was based on one perforator (Fig. 18.3).

The location of perforators around the abdomen was preoperatively determined by an ultrasound Doppler, and the design of the flap was based on the size and three-dimensional features of the wound. The flap was designed including the point where the cutaneous perforators were located (Fig. 18.4).

Flap Elevation

Schematic drawing of the flap

The flap was elevated from lateral to medial on the surface of the deep fascia. When elevation reaches the lateral border of the rectus sheath, attention should be paid to preserve the perforators as much as possible, and care is taken to dissect out the superficial epigastric vein to its origin to augment venous outflow if necessary. The biggest perforator is chosen as the vascular pedicle, and the anterior rectus sheath is incised about 1 mm around the chosen perforator. Then the sheath is incised longitudinally without injuring the rectus muscle. The muscle is separated in the direction of the fibers, and the joining of the perforator to a branch of the deep inferior epigastric vessels is confirmed. Next step is the key of the whole operation; microsurgical instruments were required to use for making deep intramuscular separation along the perforator vessels under a microscope (10×) until the trunk of the inferior epigastric vessels, and then enter from the outer rectus abdominis and isolate the inferior epigastric vessels. A second perforator could be included into the flap if it was located on the same row and near each other. Once the adequacy of the pedicle is ascertained, other perforators are coagulated and severed. More than two perforators need to be dissected when harvesting bilobed flap or large area flap which two perforators are not enough to supply (Fig. 18.5).

The pedicle is dissected in accordance with its required length, try best to preserve the nerves of the rectus muscle (Fig. 18.6).

Flap Transfer (Fig. 18.7)

The inferior epigastric artery was anastomosed to the dorsal artery of the foot in an end-to-end pattern. The two concomitant veins were anastomosed (Fig. 18.8).

The rectus muscle is sutured, a drain inserted, and the anterior rectus sheath closed. Finally, the skin is approximated and sutured after mobilization of the edges (Fig. 18.9).

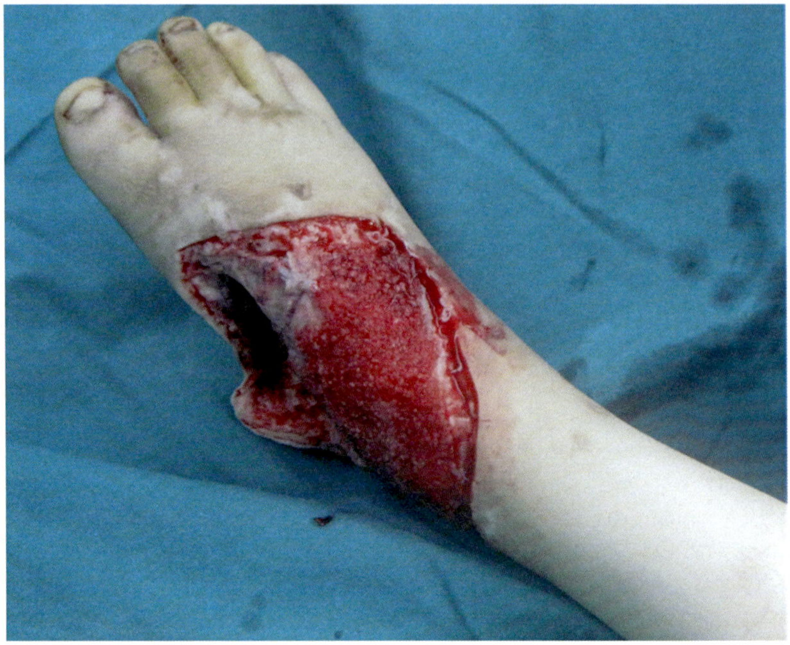

Fig. 18.2 Preoperative view (The case is offered by Professor Jun Liu and Dr. Xiaodan Xia, Hand Surgical Centre, Nanhua Hospital, Nanhua University, Henyang, China)

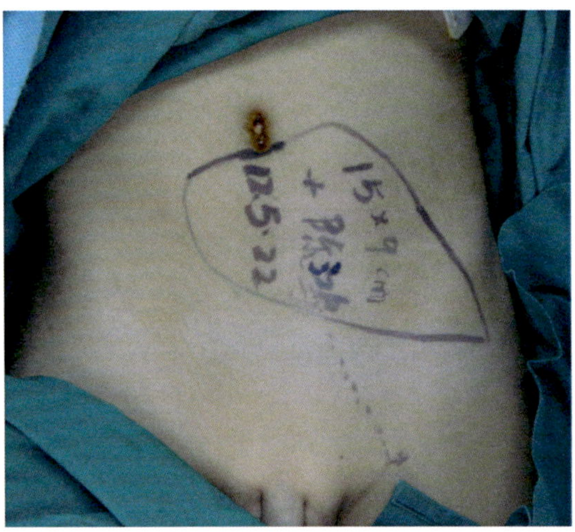

Fig. 18.3 Flap design

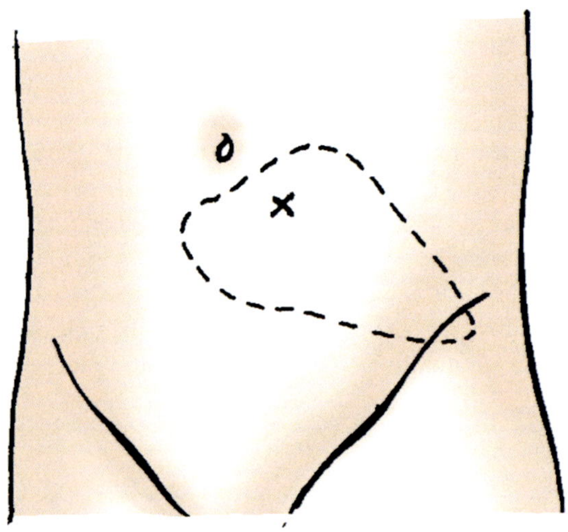

Fig. 18.4 Schematic drawing of the flap design

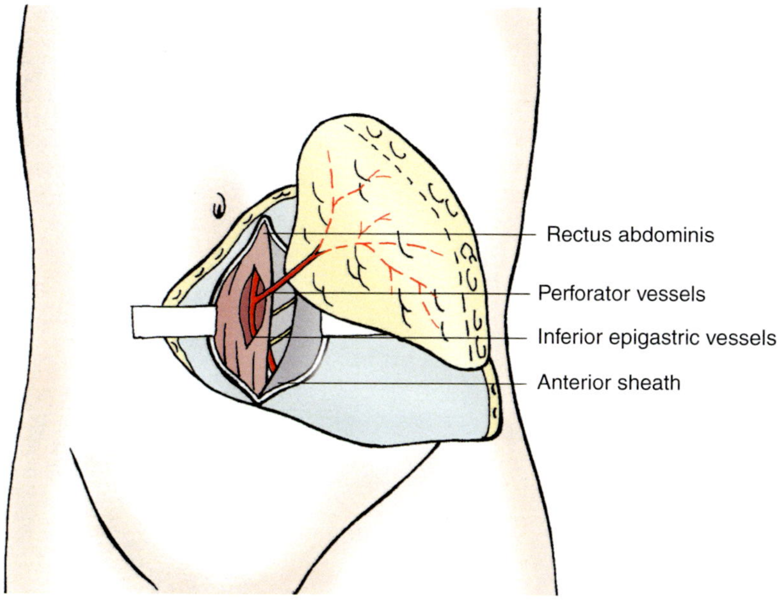

Fig. 18.5 Pedicle dissection

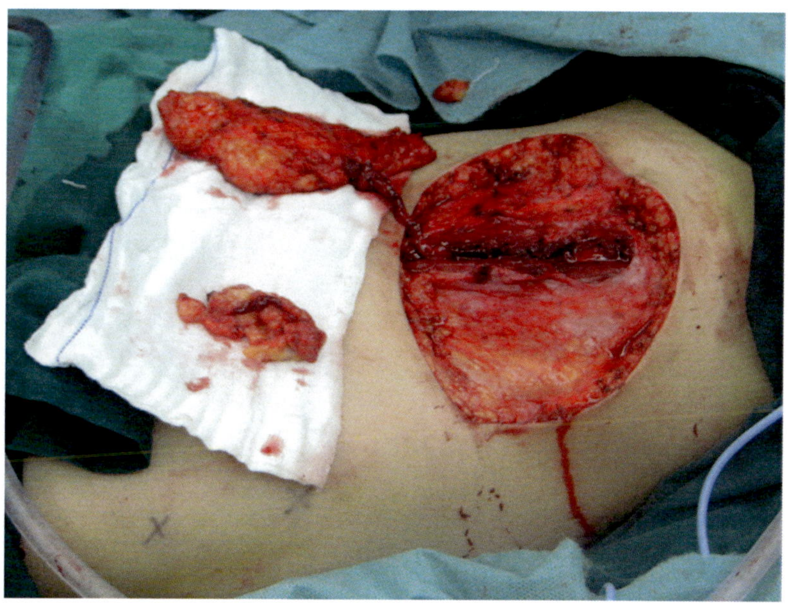

Fig. 18.6 Flap elevation

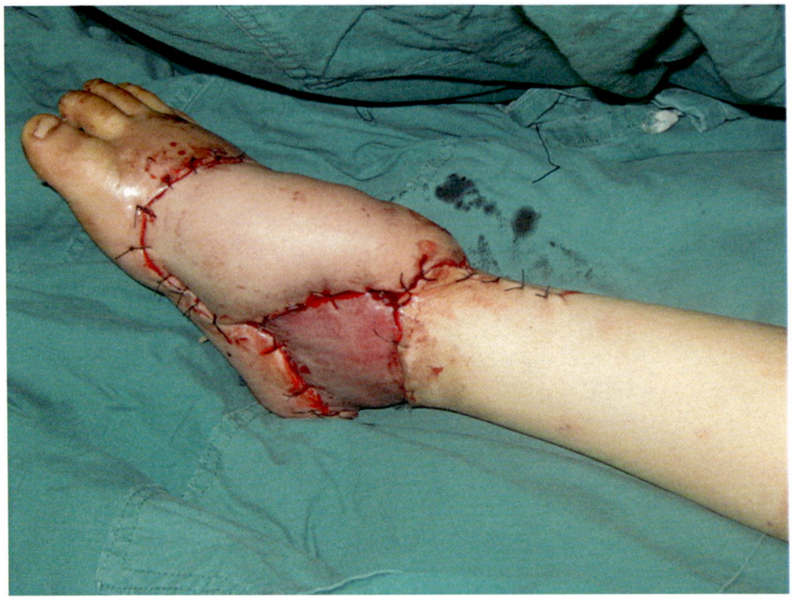

Fig. 18.7 Postoperative view

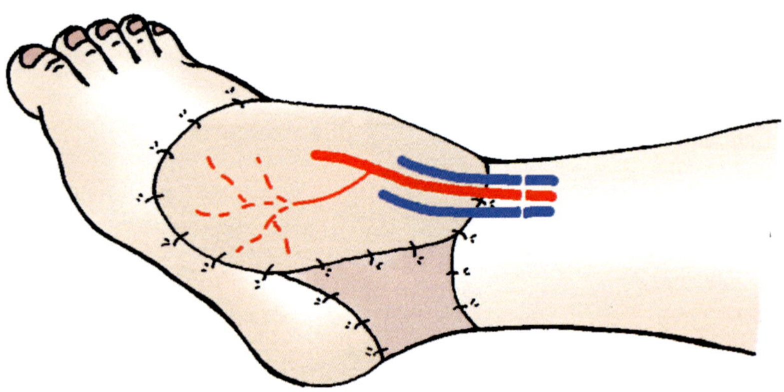

Fig. 18.8 Rebuilding the blood supply

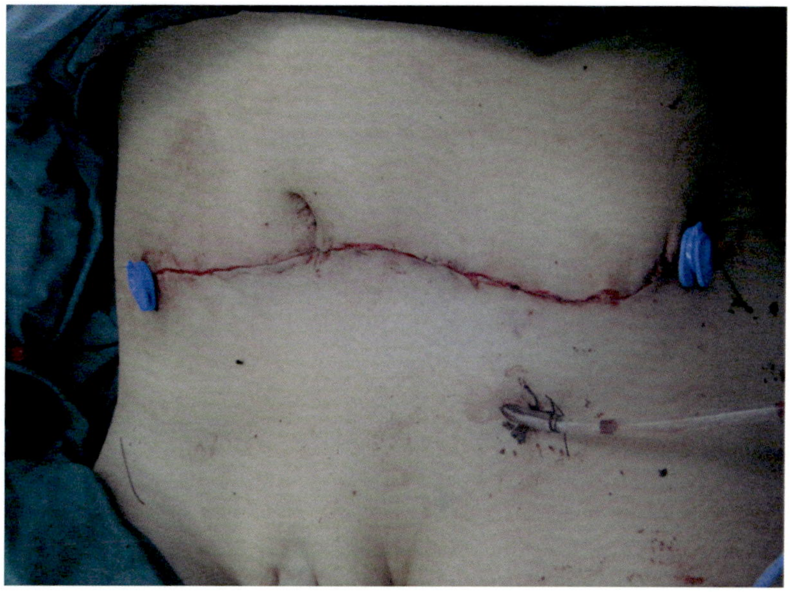

Fig. 18.9 Donor-site appearance

Pearls

There are many advantages of DIEP flaps. Apart from better cosmesis of the skin and soft tissue, which has especially led to a marked decrease in hernia rate, there is no sacrifice of the abdominal musculature, and in comparison with the free TRAM flap, the DIEP flap provides a significantly longer pedicle, allowing tension-free anastomoses, provides reliable and safe vascular supply, has versatility of its design, and is suitable for any type of head, neck, and extremity defect. In addition, the donor site can be closed as a linear scar with direct repair of the rectus sheath, and it can be done with the patient in a supine position, allowing 2 surgical teams to operate comfortably at the same time.

By including the sensate branch of the segmental nerve, which runs along with the perforating vessel, sensory nerve repair in perforator flaps is possible.

Pitfalls

Preoperative mapping of the main perforator using an audible Doppler can facilitate planning the flap design.

The subcutaneous layer should be incised and dissected from lateral toward the umbilicus. This makes dissection easier, and it is less likely that a perforator is missed.

Uplifting the deep inferior epigastric artery helps localize side branches, which must be carefully clipped. The posterior rectus sheath must not be opened.

The deep superior epigastric artery can also be used as the source vessel.

The branches of the periumbilical perforators radiate in any direction of the abdominal skin, thus making it possible to harvest flaps with virtually any orientation.

References

1. Koshima I, Soeda S. Inferior epigastric artery skin flaps without rectus abdominis muscle. Br J Plast Surg. 1989;42(6):645–8.
2. Acosta R, Smit JM, Audolfsson T, et al. A clinical review of 9 years of free perforator flap breast reconstructions: an analysis of 675 flaps and the influence of new techniques on clinical practice. J Reconstr Microsurg. 2011;27(2):91–8.
3. Allen RJ, Treece P. Deep inferior epigastric perforator flap for breast reconstruction. Ann Plast Surg. 1994; 32(1):32–8.
4. Gill PS, Hunt JP, Guerra AB, et al. A 10-year retrospective review of 758 DIEP flaps for breast reconstruction. Plast Reconstr Surg. 2004;113(4):1153–60.
5. Masia J, Sommario M, Cervelli D, Vega C, Leon X, Pons G. Extended deep inferior epigastric artery perforator flap for head and neck reconstruction: a clinical experience with 100 patients. Head Neck. 2011; 33(9):1328–34.
6. Santanelli F, Paolini G, Renzi L, Persechino S. Preliminary experience in reconstruction of the vulva using the pedicled vertical deep inferior epigastric perforator flap. Plast Reconstr Surg. 2007;120(1): 182–6.
7. Shafighi M, Constantinescu MA, Huemer GM, et al. The extended diep flap: extending the possibilities for breast reconstruction with tissue from the lower abdomen. Microsurgery. 2013;33(1):24–31.
8. Tang J, Fang T, Song D, Liang J, Yu F, Wang C. Free deep inferior epigastric artery perforator flap for reconstruction of soft-tissue defects in extremities of children. Microsurgery. 2013;16(2):167–71.
9. Venkat R, Lee JC, Rad AN, Manahan MA, Rosson GD. Bilateral autologous breast reconstruction with deep inferior epigastric artery perforator flaps: review of a single surgeon's early experience. Microsurgery. 2012;32(4):275–80.
10. Koshima I, Inagawa K, Urushibara K, Moriguchi T. Paraumbilical perforator flap without deep inferior epigastric vessels. Plast Reconstr Surg. 1998;102(4): 1052–7.
11. Sekido M, Yamamoto Y, Makino S. Maxillary reconstruction using a free deep inferior epigastric perforator (DIEP) flap combined with vascularised costal cartilages. J Plast Reconstr Aesthet Surg JPRAS. 2006;59(12):1350–4.
12. Tan O. Versatility of the vertical designed deep inferior epigastric perforator flap. Microsurgery. 2009; 29(4):282–6.
13. Yano T, Sakuraba M, Asano T, Sarukawa S. Head and neck reconstruction with the deep inferior epigastric perforator flap: a report of two cases. Microsurgery. 2009;29(4):287–92.

19 Anterolateral Thigh Perforator Flap

When Song et al. published their paper in 1984 on the thigh as a donor site for three new flaps with the anterolateral thigh, they closely fulfilled all the characteristics of a perforator flap [1].

After the first description by Song, it took several years until this flap became popular for different reconstructive purposes. With different focuses on the variety and shapes possible when using the conventional technique, a great number of clinical series with many different soft tissue reconstructions have been reported since the early 1990s [2–24].

19.1 Vascular Anatomy

After it arises from the lateral circumflex femoral artery, the descending branch reaches the medial rim of the vastus lateralis muscle in its proximal segment and courses distally to communicate with the superior genicular artery (Fig. 19.1).

Apart from the blood supply to the vastus lateralis muscle, the descending branch divides into the myo- or septocutaneous branches, giving the anatomical basis of the myocutaneous vastus lateralis or septocutaneous anterolateral thigh perforator flap.

C. Hou et al., *Surgical Atlas of Perforator Flaps: A Microsurgical Dissection Technique*,
DOI 10.1007/978-94-017-9834-1_19,

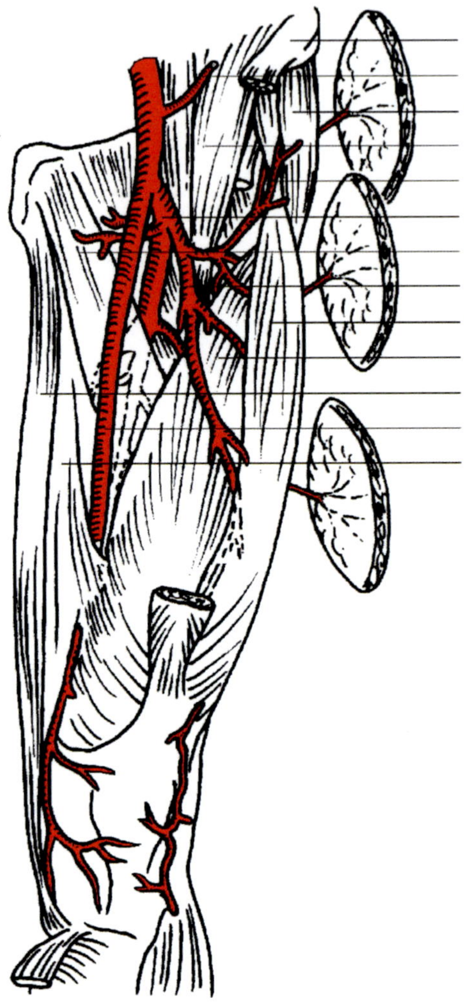

Fig. 19.1 Vascular anatomy of the descending branch of the lateral circumflex femoral artery

19.2 Illustrative Case

A 29-year-old man was struck by a motor vehicle, sustaining an avulsion injury of his left dorsum foot with tibial shaft fracture. The soft tissue defect measured 16.0 cm × 9.0 cm after thorough debridement.

Flap Design (Fig. 19.3)

The perforators can be found a few centimeters proximal to the midpoint of the interconnection between the anterior superior iliac spine and the lateral rim of the patella (Fig. 19.4).

Perforator Vessel Visualization

The skin incision is marked medial to the tensor muscle at the proximal thigh and straight above the rectus muscle toward the knee. Using magnifying loupe, these myocutaneous perforators become visible, entering the muscle along its undersurface at the anterior muscle rim (Fig. 19.5).

Flap Elevation (Fig. 19.6)

The rectus femoris and vastus lateralis muscles are bluntly separated from each other, and by retracting the rectus femoris muscle medially, the descending branch of the circumflex femoral artery with its two comitant veins becomes visible.

The myocutaneous perforator is followed through the vastus lateralis muscle.

Small side branches to the muscle are ligated or clipped, and the perforator is finally isolated with only a very small muscle cuff around it.

The skin paddle, which can now be designed in its final form, is raised completely (Fig. 19.7).

Flap Transfer and Insetting

Flap raising is finished with further dissection of the perforator in the proximal direction, until the descending branch of the lateral circumflex femoral artery is reached. The flap is now ready for microvascular transplantation (Fig. 19.8). The descending branch vessels were anastomosed with the anterior tibial vessels (A:V = 1:2) (Fig. 19.9).

The donor site was closed directly (Fig. 19.10).

Follow-Up

After rehabilitation, the patient was able to walk and climb stairs without external support 14 months postoperatively. The gait function was acceptable (Fig. 19.11).

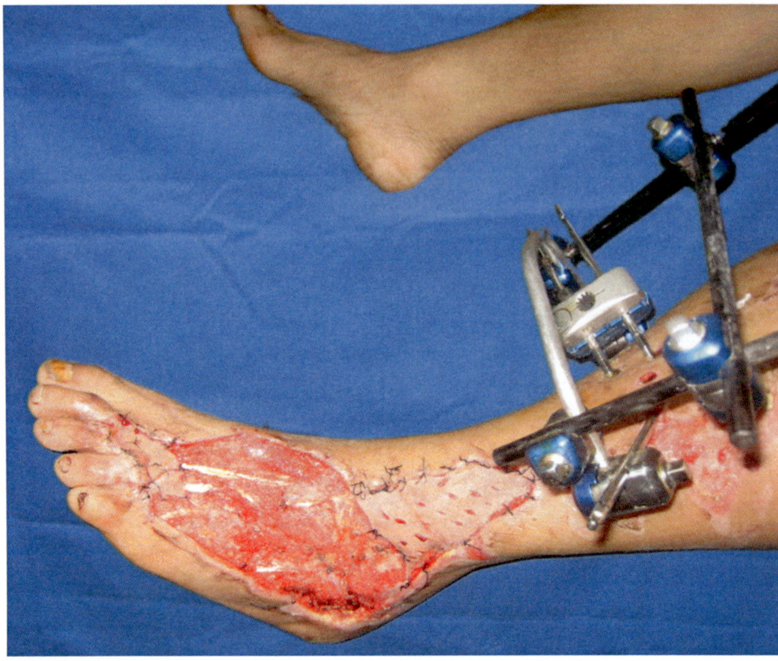

Fig. 19.2 Preoperative view

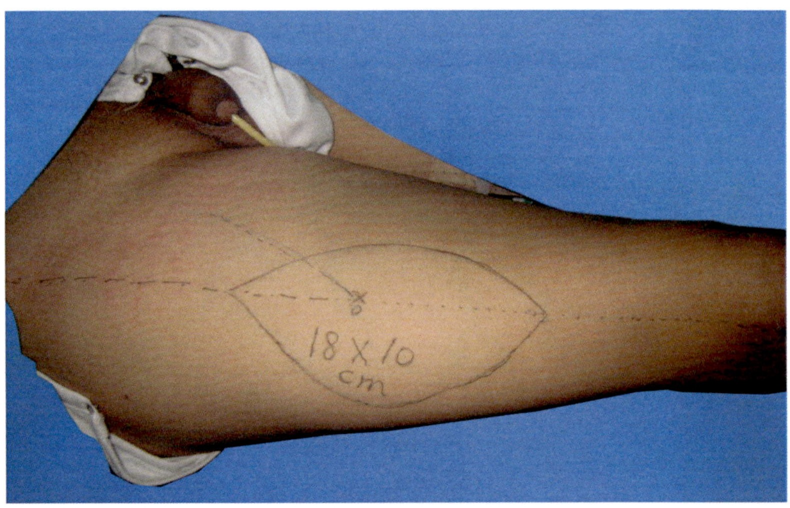

Fig. 19.3 Flap design

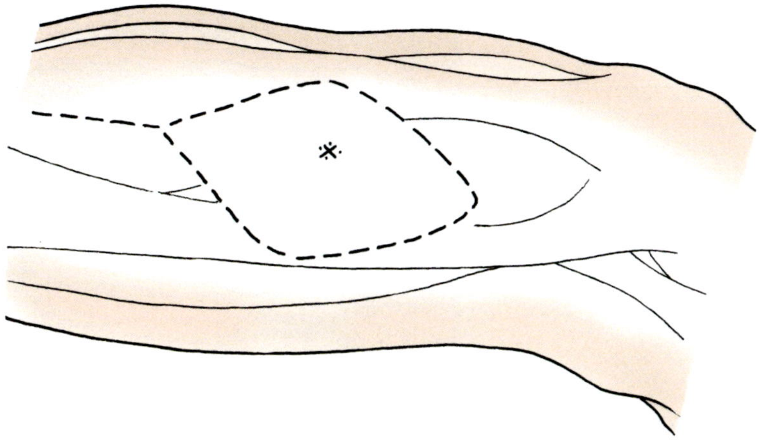

Fig. 19.4 Schematic drawing of the flap design

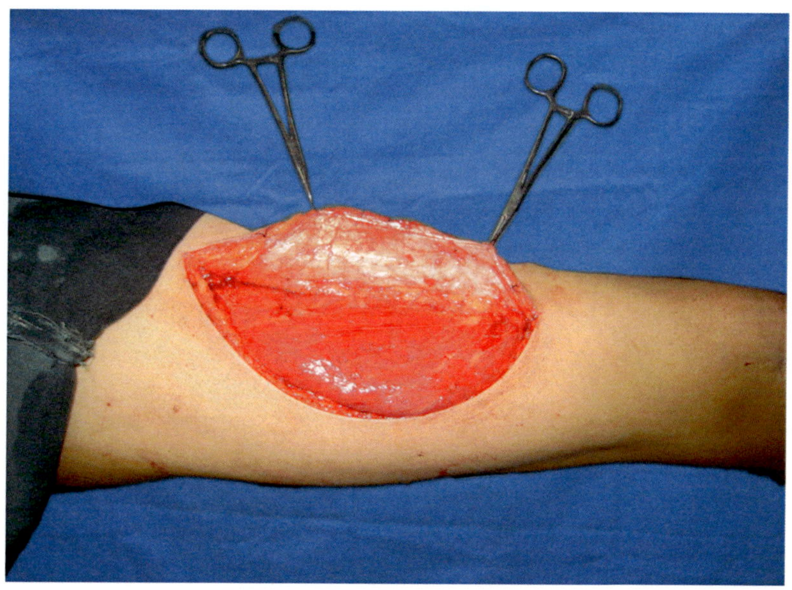

Fig. 19.5 Perforator vessel visualization

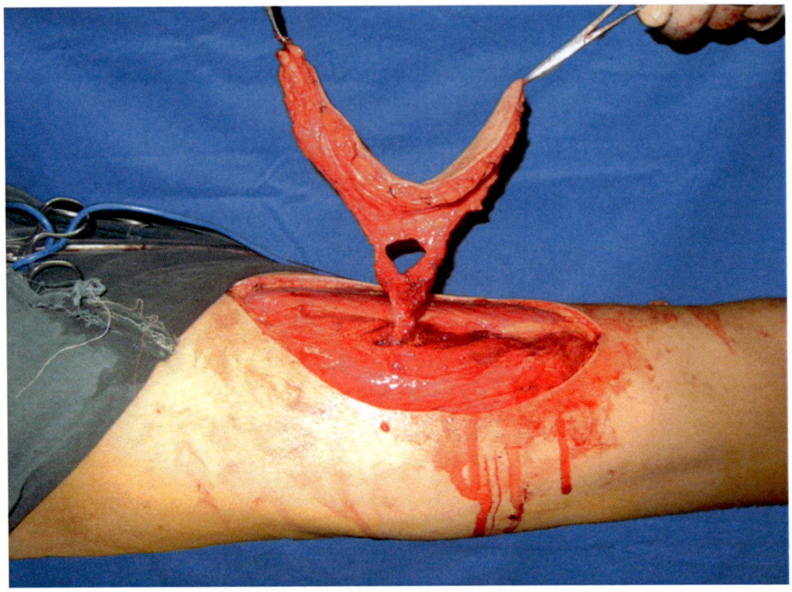

Fig. 19.6 Flap elevation

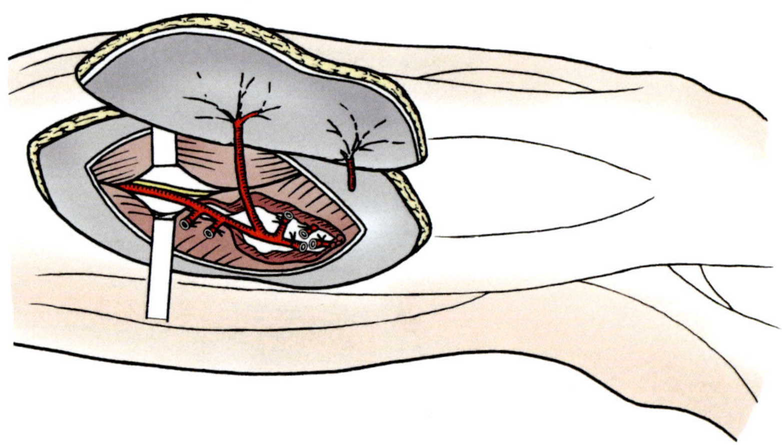

Fig. 19.7 Schematic drawing of the flap elevation

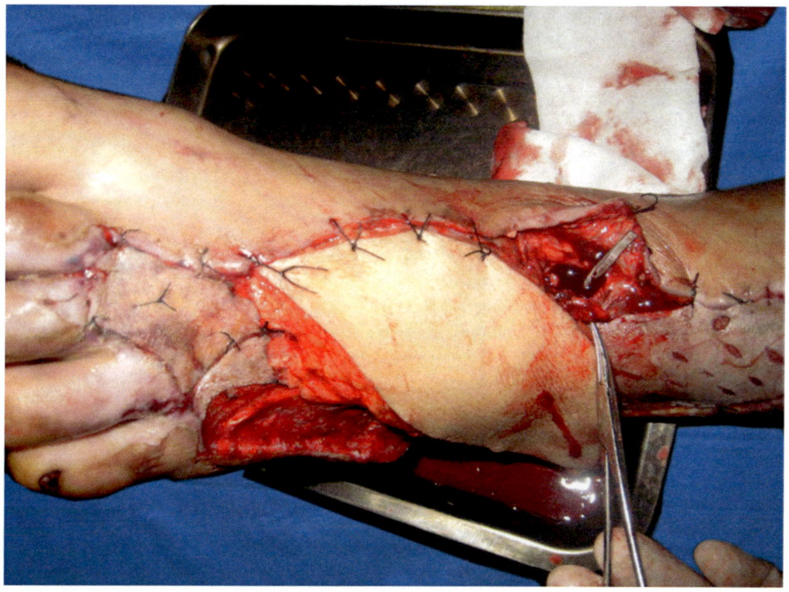

Fig. 19.8 Flap transfer and insetting

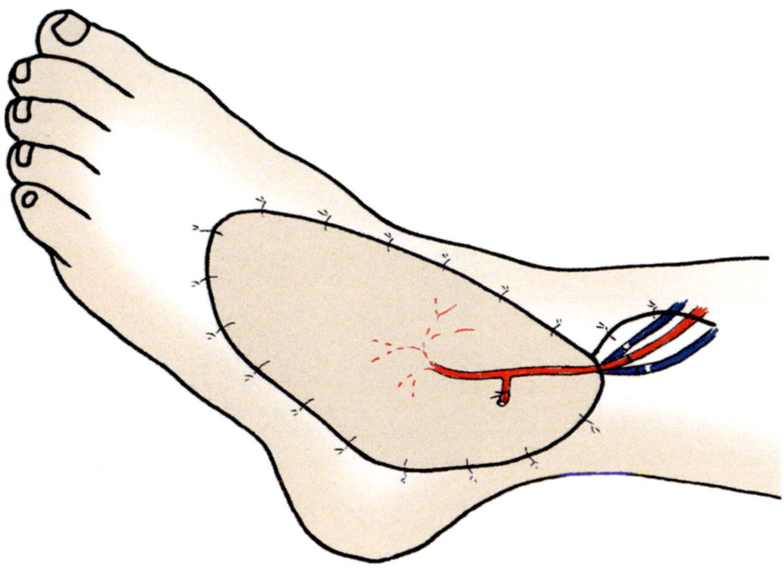

Fig. 19.9 Rebuilding the blood supply of the flap

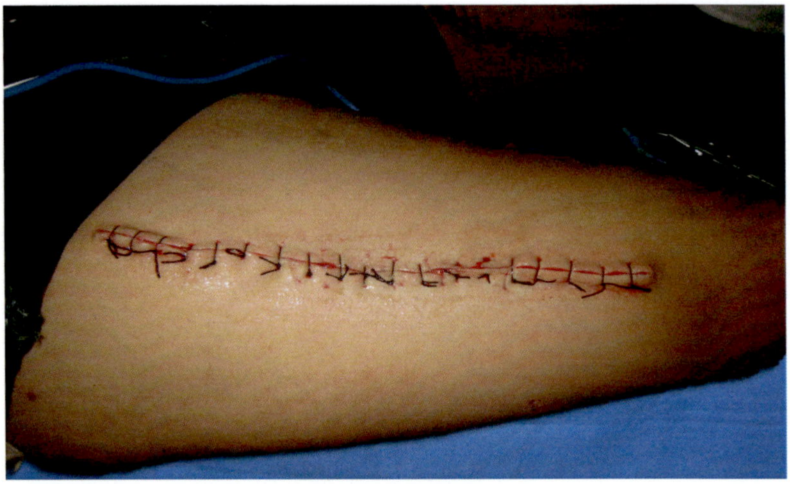

Fig. 19.10 The appearance of the donor site

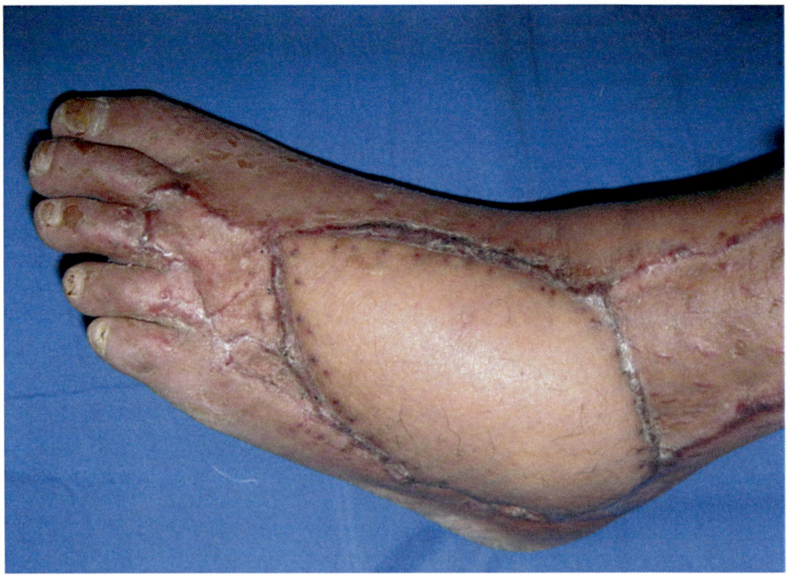

Fig. 19.11 Follow-up

Pearls

Vascular anatomy of the cutaneous perforators of the lateral thigh gives a suitable basis for primary flap thinning.

Pitfalls

Preoperative evaluation of the perforators should be performed using a Doppler probe by carefully auscultating the skin in the region of the intermuscular septum and over the medial parts of the vastus lateralis muscle.

The skin paddle of the ALT perforator flap depends completely on the location of the perforator selected for the flap. Thus, the definite design of the flap cannot be determined before a useful perforator shows that a strong pulsation has been exposed.

The skin incision to expose the main perforating vessel should not be outlined lateral to the rectus femoris muscle, because this will lead to injury of the intermuscular septum.

To determine the appropriate vein for anastomosis, venous return should be checked if possible before the pedicle is completely transected.

References

1. Song YG, Chen GZ, Song YL. The free thigh flap: a new free flap concept based on the septocutaneous artery. Br J Plast Surg. 1984;37(2):149–59.
2. Ao M, Nagase Y, Mae O, Namba Y. Reconstruction of posttraumatic defects of the foot by flow-through anterolateral or anteromedial thigh flaps with preservation of posterior tibial vessels. Ann Plast Surg. 1997;38(6):598–603.
3. Ji Y, Li T, Shamburger S, Jin J, Lineaweaver WC, Zhang F. Microsurgical anterolateral thigh fasciocutaneous flap for facial contour correction in patients with hemifacial microsomia. Microsurgery. 2002;22(1):34–8.
4. Koshima I, Kawada S, Etoh H, Kawamura S, Moriguchi T, Sonoh H. Flow-through anterior thigh flaps for one-stage reconstruction of soft-tissue defects and revascularization of ischemic extremities. Plast Reconstr Surg. 1995;95(2):252–60.
5. Gravvanis A, Lo S, Shirley R. Aesthetic restoration of Poland's syndrome in a male patient using free anterolateral thigh perforator flap as autologous filler. Microsurgery. 2009;29(6):490–4.
6. Hsieh CH, Yang CC, Kuo YR, Tsai HH, Jeng SF. Free anterolateral thigh adipofascial perforator flap. Plast Reconstr Surg. 2003;112(4):976–82.
7. Wolff KD, Kesting M, Loffelbein D, Holzle F. Perforator-based anterolateral thigh adipofascial or dermal fat flaps for facial contour augmentation. J Reconstr Microsurg. 2007;23(8):497–503.
8. Gedebou TM, Wei FC, Lin CH. Clinical experience of 1284 free anterolateral thigh flaps. Handchirurgie Mikrochirurgie plastische Chirurgie Organ der Deutschsprachigen Arbeitsgemeinschaft fur Handchirurgie Organ der Deutschsprachigen Arbeitsgemeinschaft fur Mikrochirurgie der Peripheren Nerven und Gefasse. 2002;34(4):239–44.
9. Koshima I, Yamamoto H, Hosoda M, Moriguchi T, Orita Y, Nagayama H. Free combined composite flaps using the lateral circumflex femoral system for repair of massive defects of the head and neck regions: an introduction to the chimeric flap principle. Plast Reconstr Surg. 1993;92(3):411–20.
10. Shieh SJ, Chiu HY, Yu JC, Pan SC, Tsai ST, Shen CL. Free anterolateral thigh flap for reconstruction of head and neck defects following cancer ablation. Plast Reconstr Surg. 2000;105(7):2349–57; discussion 2358–2360.
11. Wei FC, Jain V, Celik N, Chen HC, Chuang DC, Lin CH. Have we found an ideal soft-tissue flap? An experience with 672 anterolateral thigh flaps. Plast Reconstr Surg. 2002;109(7):2219–26; discussion 2227–2230.
12. Zhou G, Qiao Q, Chen GY, Ling YC, Swift R. Clinical experience and surgical anatomy of 32 free anterolateral thigh flap transplantations. Br J Plast Surg. 1991;44(2):91–6.
13. Heller F, Hsu CM, Chuang CC, Wei KC, Wei FC. Anterolateral thigh fasciocutaneous flap for simultaneous reconstruction of refractory scalp and dural defects. Report of two cases. J Neurosurg. 2004;100(6):1094–7.
14. Kimura N, Satoh K. Consideration of a thin flap as an entity and clinical applications of the thin anterolateral thigh flap. Plast Reconstr Surg. 1996;97(5):985–92.
15. Kimura N, Satoh K, Hasumi T, Ostuka T. Clinical application of the free thin anterolateral thigh flap in 31 consecutive patients. Plast Reconstr Surg. 2001;108(5):1197–208; discussion 1209–1110.
16. Wolff KD, Plath T, Hoffmeister B. Primary thinning of the myocutaneous vastus lateralis flap. Int J Oral Maxillofac Surg. 2000;29(4):272–6.
17. Wolff KD, Plath T, Frege J, Hoffmeister B. [Primary thinning and de-epithelialization of microsurgical transplants from the lateral thigh]. Mund Kiefer und Gesichtschirurgie MKG. 2000;4(2):88–94.
18. Chen HC, Tang YB. Anterolateral thigh flap: an ideal soft tissue flap. Clin Plast Surg. 2003;30(3):383–401.

19. Demirkan F, Chen HC, Wei FC, et al. The versatile anterolateral thigh flap: a musculocutaneous flap in disguise in head and neck reconstruction. Br J Plast Surg. 2000;53(1):30–6.
20. Kimata Y, Uchiyama K, Sekido M, et al. Anterolateral thigh flap for abdominal wall reconstruction. Plast Reconstr Surg. 1999;103(4):1191–7.
21. Posch NA, Mureau MA, Flood SJ, Hofer SO. The combined free partial vastus lateralis with anterolateral thigh perforator flap reconstruction of extensive composite defects. Br J Plast Surg. 2005;58(8):1095–103.
22. Wolff KD. Indications for the vastus lateralis flap in oral and maxillofacial surgery. Br J Oral Maxillofac Surg. 1998;36(5):358–64.
23. Wolff KD, Metelmann HR. Applications of the lateral vastus muscle flap. Int J Oral Maxillofac Surg. 1992; 21(4):215–8.
24. Wolff KD, Dienemann D, Hoffmeister B. Intraoral defect coverage with muscle flaps. J Oral Maxillofac Surg Off J Am Assoc Oral Maxillofac Surg. 1995; 53(6):680–5; discussion 686.

20 Vastus Medialis Perforator Flap

The anatomical basis and the clinical application of the vastus medialis perforator flap was firstly reported by Zheng and Lin [1].

20.1 Vascular Anatomy

A large muscular artery, named the medial vastus medialis artery, is given off from the superficial femoral artery at the tip of the femoral triangle, which then travels laterally downward along the muscle fibers after entering the muscle and anastomoses with the rete patellae when it reaches the knee joint. The site of the first musculocutaneous perforator is relatively constant, whose piercing point into the fascia can be located around the midpoint of the surface projection line (a line drawn from the junction of the middle and lower thirds of the line between the midpoint of the inguinal groove and the medial femoral condyle to the midpoint of the upper margin of the patella) of the medial vastus medialis artery (Fig. 20.1).

C. Hou et al., *Surgical Atlas of Perforator Flaps: A Microsurgical Dissection Technique*,
DOI 10.1007/978-94-017-9834-1_20,

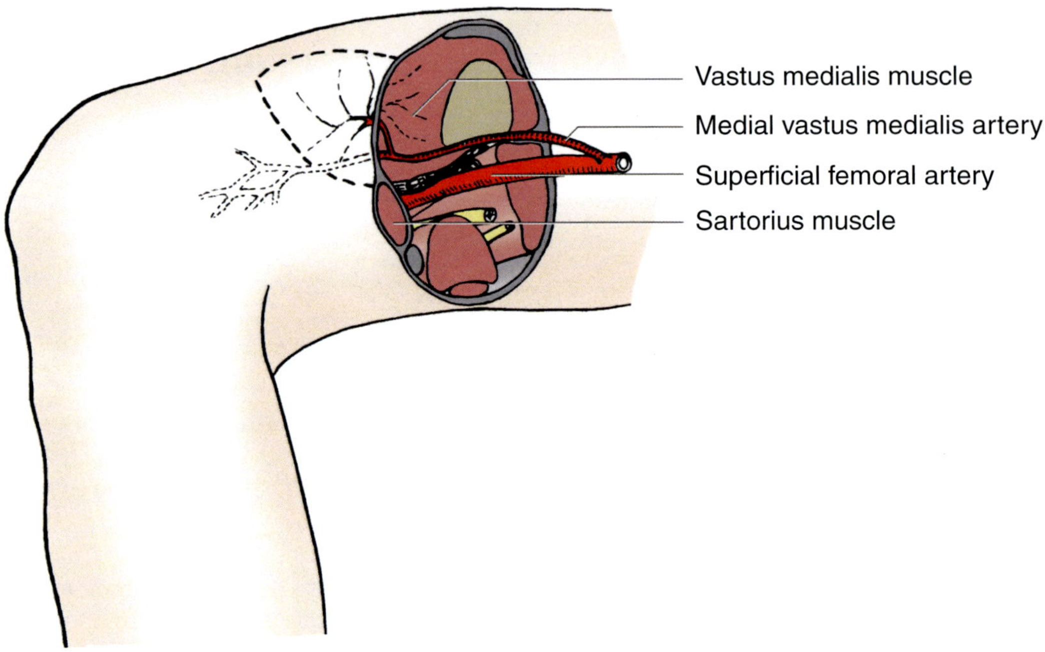

Fig. 20.1 Vascular anatomy of the medial vastus medialis artery

20.2 Illustrative Case

A 28-year-old female sustained a soft tissue defect at the anterior aspect of the right knee in a traffic accident.

During operation, the wound was radically debrided at first, resulting in a defect measuring 5.0×3.3 cm (Fig. 20.2).

Flap Design

After debridement, the patient was positioned with the hip flexed and the affected limb slightly abducted and rotated laterally. A handheld Doppler probe was regularly employed to locate the site of the perforator(s) preoperatively. The axial line was defined as the surface projection line of the medial vastus medialis artery, which was detailed above (Fig. 20.3). A template of the flap was outlined at the donor site, according to the preoperative design (Fig. 20.4).

Flap Elevation

An incision was first made at the lateral superior border of the flap deep down to the layer underneath the fascia lata (Fig. 20.5), and dissection was then carried out in a proximal-to-distal direction until the musculocutaneous perforator(s) site was encountered (Fig. 20.6).

Flap Transfer

Meticulous retrograde (distal-to-proximal direction) intramuscular dissection was performed to trace the perforator(s) to the medial vastus medialis artery. A small muscular cuff should be preserved around the perforator(s) to avoid damage to them. When designed as a proximally based flap, the medial vastus medialis artery was ligated and divided proximally to the musculocutaneous perforator(s) and vice versa; dissection was performed until sufficient length of the vascular pedicle was obtained (Fig. 20.7).

Flap Insetting

The flap was then transposed and inset into the recipient site. The donor site was closed primarily (Fig. 20.8).

The color of the flaps in the patient was similar to the surrounding tissue; the patient resumed his daily activities (Fig. 20.9).

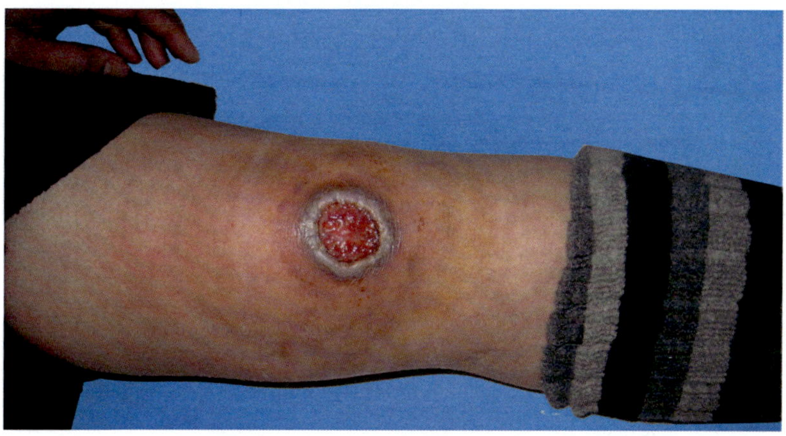

Fig. 20.2 Preoperative view

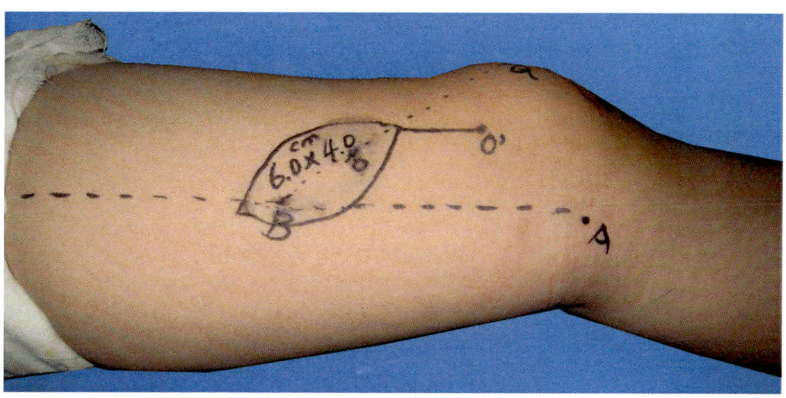

Fig. 20.3 Flap design

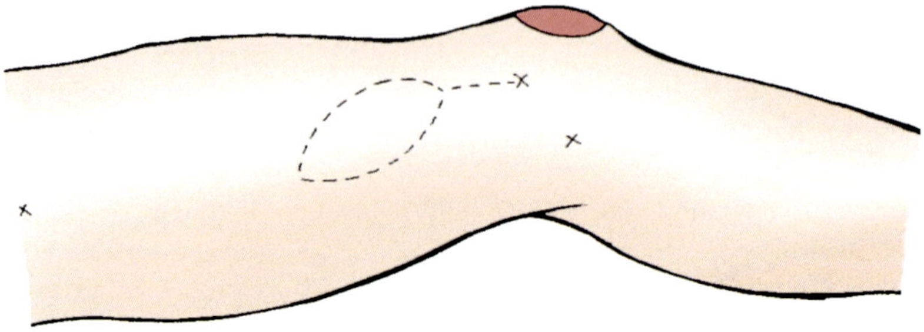

Fig. 20.4 Schematic drawing of the flap design

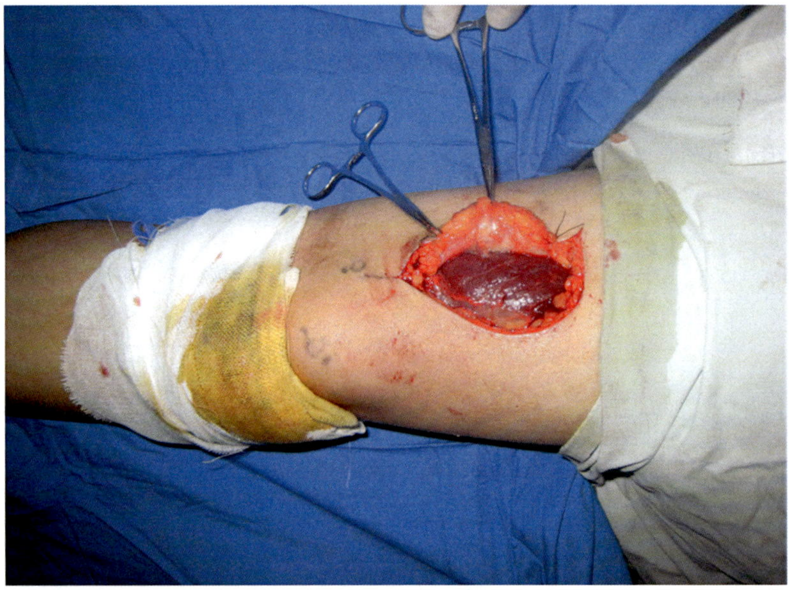

Fig. 20.5 Flap elevation

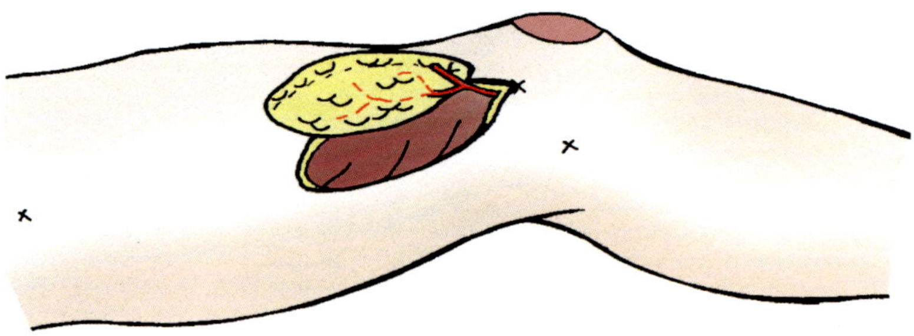

Fig. 20.6 Schematic drawing of the flap

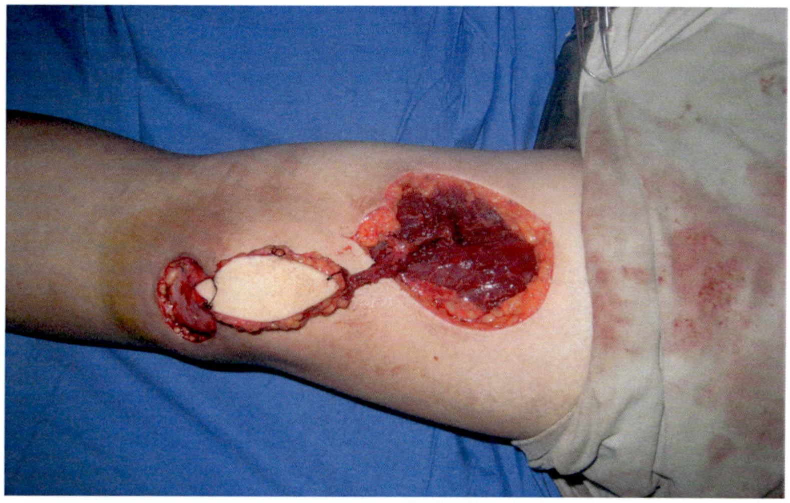

Fig. 20.7 Flap transfer

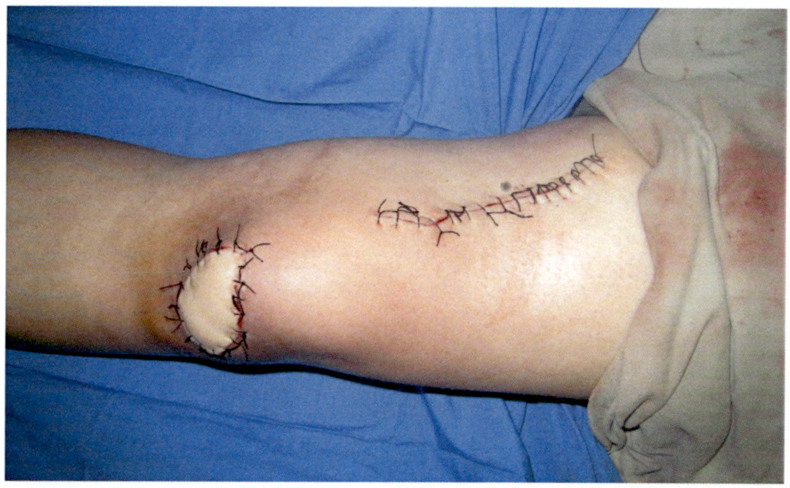

Fig. 20.8 Flap insetting

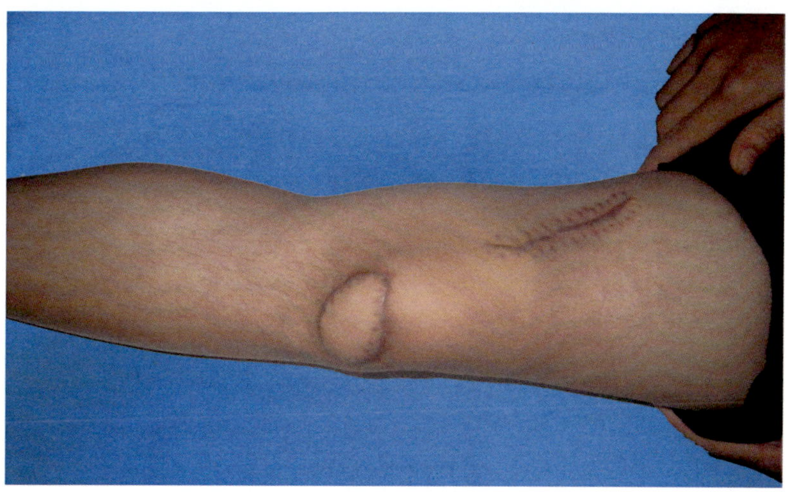

Fig. 20.9 Follow-up

Pearls

The donor site can be closed primarily if the width of the flap does not exceed 9 cm, and the scar can be concealed even in summer by wearing a parallel-knee short pant.

What is more, vessels originate from the vastus medialis to the quadriceps femoris tendon, supplying the region of the tendon adjacent to the vastus medialis insertion of the tendon, implying that it has the potential to be harvested containing part of the vascularized quadriceps femoris tendon as a composite perforator flap for reconstruction of extension mechanism of the knee when it is impaired.

By anastomosing the intermediate cutaneous nerve of the thigh with a nerve in the recipient site, the flap has the potential to be made sensate.

Pitfalls

If a larger flap is to be harvested, it is recommended to make a small modification to change the axis of the flap to the surface projection line of the intermediate cutaneous nerve of the thigh (the line connecting the midpoint of the inguinal groove with the medial femoral condyle) so that distal perfusion of blood can be strengthened through a lower-resistance longitudinal nutrient vascular plexus (true anastomoses) of the cutaneous nerve.

Reference

1. Zheng HP, Lin J, Zhuang YH, Zhang FH. Convenient coverage of soft-tissue defects around the knee by the pedicled vastus medialis perforator flap. J Plast Reconstr Aesthet Surg. 2012;65(9):1151–7.

Saphenous Artery Perforator Flap

21

In 1981, an international group of surgeons under the direction of Acland published their work on the "saphenous flap" [1–3].

21.1 Vascular Anatomy

The saphenous artery arises from the descending genicular artery. About 2 cm from its origin, the saphenous artery continues distally and pierces the roof of the adductor canal. After the artery passes through the roof of the adductor canal, it runs in the loose fascial space bounded by the sartorius muscle superficially, the adductor tendon posteriorly, and the bulging vastus medialis muscle anterolaterally.

It then courses straight down the leg in this space for 12–15 cm. In this part, it gives off early cutaneous branches that supply the large area of medial thigh skin above the knee. The cutaneous branches are given off 3–10 cm from the origin of the saphenous artery. The saphenous artery continues on its straight course, running from behind the tendon to enter the subcutaneous tissue. It supplies another large area of skin on the anterior and medial aspects of the leg below the knee (Fig. 21.1).

C. Hou et al., *Surgical Atlas of Perforator Flaps: A Microsurgical Dissection Technique*,
DOI 10.1007/978-94-017-9834-1_21,

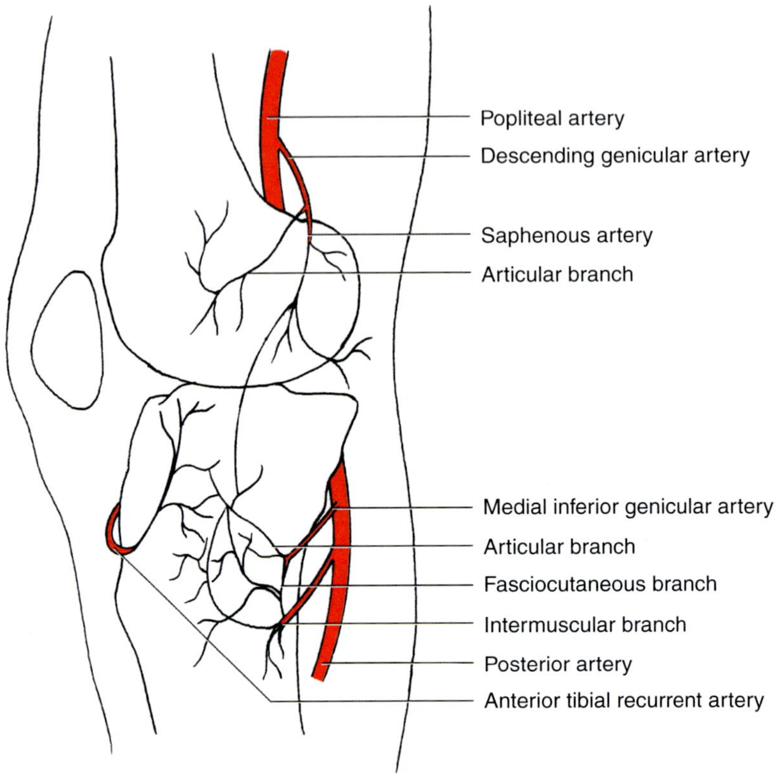

Fig. 21.1 Vascular anatomy of the saphenous artery

21.2 Illustrative Case

A 40-year-old man presented with severe scar ulcer on the popliteal space. Thirty-seven years before the patient suffered from traffic accident, early skin grafting was performed, but the ulcer occurred on the skin grafting area 5 years before (Fig. 21.2).

Flap Design

After radical debridement (Fig. 21.3), a pedicled saphenous perforator flap was designed. The key landmark for localizing the vascular pedicle is the sartorius muscle (Fig. 21.4). A line should be drawn from the anterior superior iliac spine to the medial epicondyle of the tibia, approximating the course of the muscle. The final position of the flap axis and skin paddle is determined after the position of the cutaneous perforators is confirmed (Fig. 21.5).

Either selective angiography or Doppler ultrasound assists in localizing these perforators preoperatively.

Flap Elevation

A linear incision 10 cm long is made on the middle of the medial aspect of the thigh, with its distal end 12 cm above the knee. The incision is made down to deep fascia that overlies the sartorius muscle. The subcutaneous fat is dissected off the deep fascia until the anterior border of the sartorius muscle is reached. Just anterior to the border of the sartorius muscle, the deep fascia is incised from end to end of the wound. Care is taken to identify and preserve cutaneous nerves that lie just below the fascia. The space between the vastus medialis and the sartorius muscles is then opened with finger dissection. The saphenous artery is immediately identified toward the distal end of the wound. It lies deep between the two muscles (Fig. 21.6).

Once an adequate perforator has been identified, the flap is outlined so that these branches will provide adequate circulation. The skin incision is extended anteriorly and distally to encompass these cutaneous branches. The extension of this incision forms the anterior flap margin. The width needed to cover the defect is marked, and the flap is raised anterior to posterior. Any other branches of the saphenous artery that are encountered as the flap is raised are dissected and preserved with the flap (Fig. 21.7).

Flap Transfer and Insetting

The flap was rotated 120°to cover the wound. The donor site was closed by skin grafts (Fig. 21.8).

Follow-Up

The flap survived smoothly. The texture and appearance was satisfactory (Fig. 21.9).

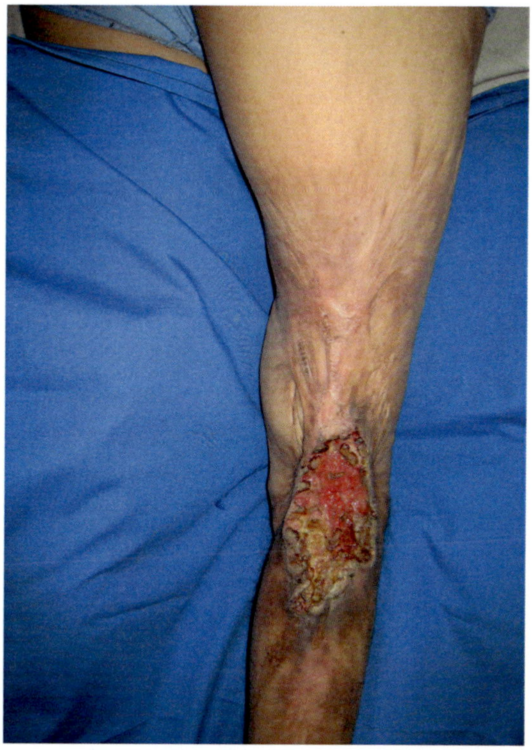

Fig. 21.2 Preoperative view

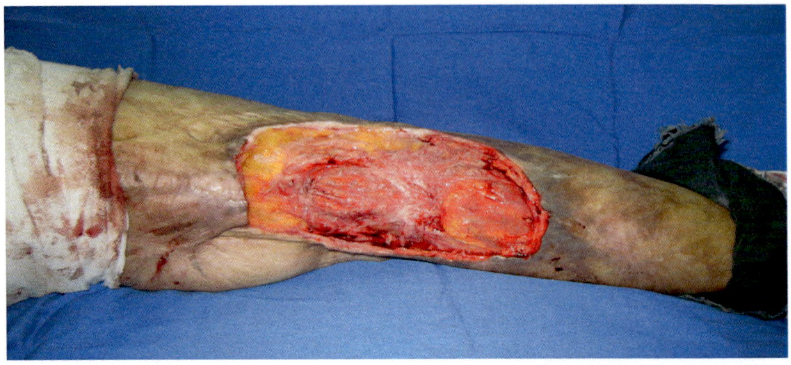

Fig. 21.3 The defect after radical debridement

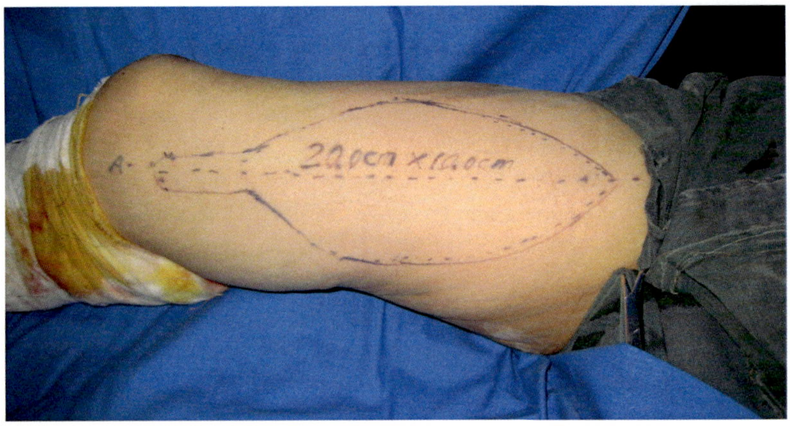

Fig. 21.4 Flap design

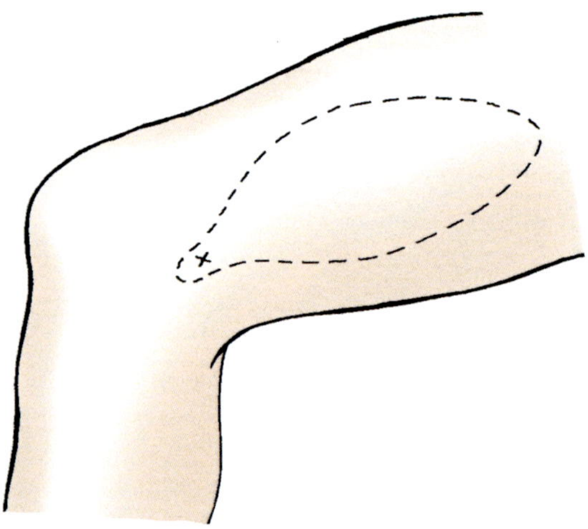

Fig. 21.5 Schematic drawing of the flap design

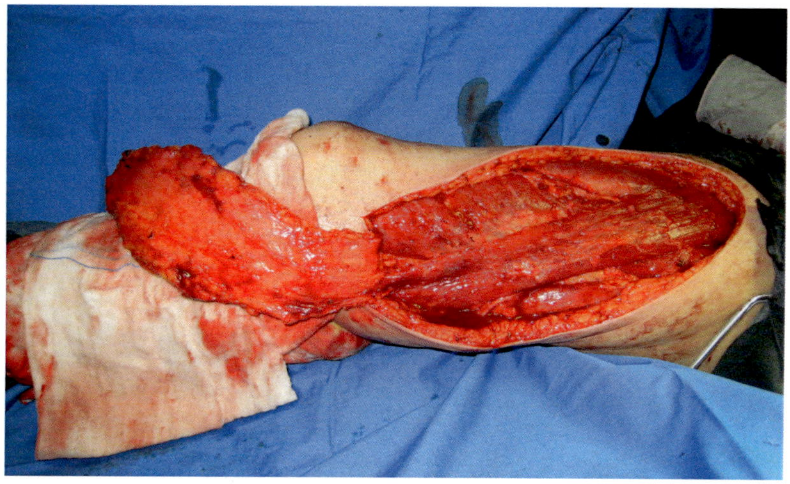

Fig. 21.6 Flap elevation

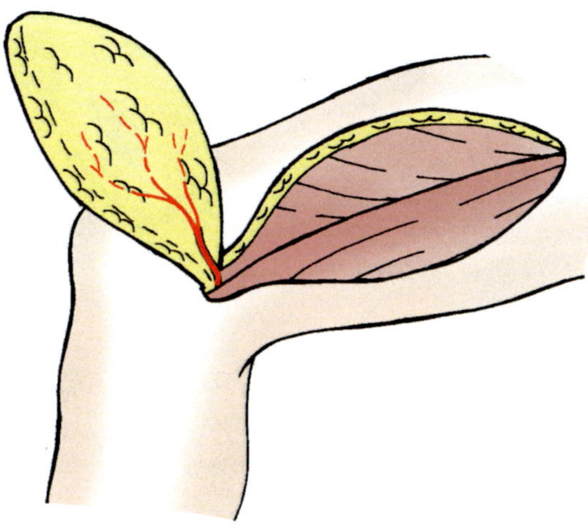

Fig. 21.7 Schematic drawing of the flap elevation

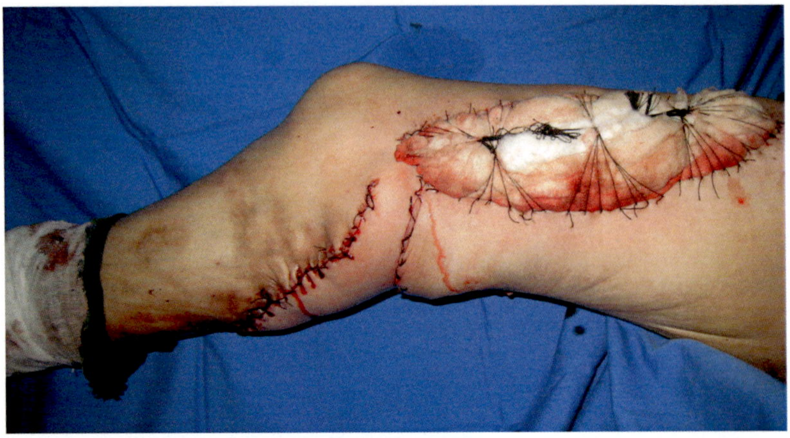

Fig. 21.8 Flap transfer and insetting

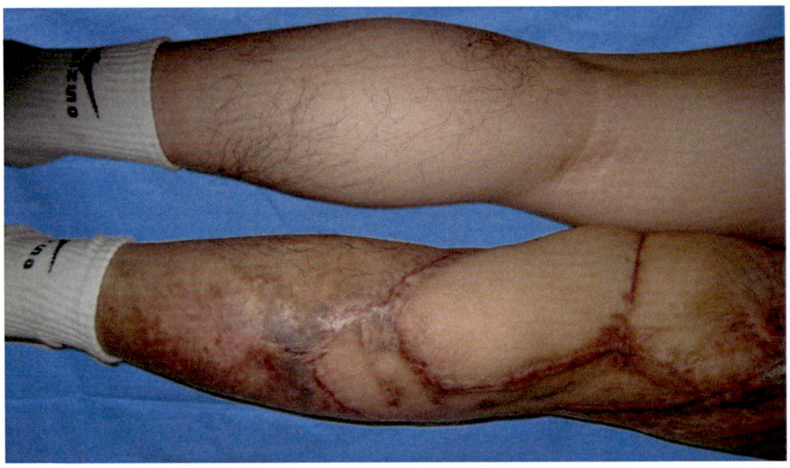

Fig. 21.9 Follow-up

Pearls

(1) As a physiological tissue flap, it has a high survival rate; (2) there is less injury to the donor site and no significant impact on the muscle function or power resulting from the partial incision of the sartorius muscle; (3) the big rotation arc of the flap enables it to repair a complex traumatic surface involving the inferior one-third of the leg, ankle, and foot, including cases of nonunion and bone defect; and (4) avoiding the fixation of the operative limb, when possible, is advantageous to participation in early functional exercise.

Pitfalls

There is significant variability with the vascular anatomy; therefore, definitive placement of the skin paddle should be avoided until the cutaneous perforators from the saphenous artery have been identified.

The descending genicular artery is absent in about 5 % of cases. Koshima et al. suggested that the flap could be salvaged in this situation by using the distal nutrient vessel from the sartorius as the basis of a musculocutaneous flap, without the need to alter the skin paddle. This situation can be avoided by using preoperative duplex ultrasound or CTA to confirm the presence of the saphenous artery before starting the flap harvest [4, 5].

References

1. Acland RD, Schusterman M, Godina M, Eder E, Taylor GI, Carlisle I. The saphenous neurovascular free flap. Plast Reconstr Surg. 1981;67(6):763–74.
2. Gao XS, Liu L, Yuan XB. [Median-knee saphenous neurovascular flap for ipsilateral or cross-leg transfer]. Zhonghua wai ke za zhi [Chin J Surg]. 1986;24(1):36–7, 63.
3. Lu KH, Luo JH, Guo SZ. [Clinical uses of the saphenous neurovascular axial skin flap in treating skin defects of the lower extremity]. Zhonghua wai ke za zhi [Chin J Surg]. 1986;24(12):762–4, 783.
4. Tsai CC, Lin SD, Lai CS, Chou CK, Lin TM. Reconstruction of the upper leg and knee with a reversed flow saphenous island flap based on the medial inferior genicular artery. Ann Plast Surg. 1995;35(5):480–4.
5. Koshima I, Endou T, Soeda S, Yamasaki M. The free or pedicled saphenous flap. Ann Plast Surg. 1988;21(4):369–74.

22 Posterior Thigh Perforator Flap

Hurwitz [1] described the first posterior thigh flap in 1980, when he used a musculocutaneous flap based on the inferior gluteal artery.

Ramirez et al. [2] reported on the posterolateral fascia lata flap, showing that it received branches from the first deep femoral perforating artery.

In 1984, Song et al. [3] documented a posterior thigh flap based on the third perforating branch of the profunda femoris artery.

In 1989, Maruyama and Iwahira [4] documented a popliteoposterior thigh fasciocutaneous island flap based on a direct branch of the popliteal artery for coverage of a knee wound.

This branch, however, was found to be inconsistent by Cormack and Lamberty [5].

In 1993, Paletta et al. [6] performed a posterior thigh flap based on the descending branch of the inferior gluteal artery to raise a posterior thigh island flap, an extended gluteal thigh flap, an ipsilateral pedicled thigh flap, and a local rotation flap.

In 1996, Lambert et al. [7] performed a posterior thigh fasciocutaneous flap based distally on a branch from the popliteal artery.

22.1 Vascular Anatomy

The largest part of the posterior thigh skin territory is supplied by the profunda femoris artery [5, 8], mostly by the first and second profunda femoris perforating arteries [9].

The first perforating branch of the profunda femoris artery arises superior to the adductor brevis muscle and pierces the adductor magnus muscle 2–4 cm inferior to the ischial tuberosity.

The third perforating branch of the profunda femoris artery arises inferior to the adductor brevis muscle and deep to the tendon of the adductor longus muscle. The vessel passes posteriorly through the adductor magnus muscle and the short head of the biceps femoris muscle and then sends branches to the vastus lateralis muscle. The third perforating branch ultimately gives off the branch that passes along the lateral intermuscular septum to supply the lateral thigh skin and the posterolateral thigh musculature. After this branch supplies the biceps femoris muscle, it also perforates the deep fascia to supply the skin of the median aspect of the posterior thigh, the pedicle of which ranges in length from 5 [3] to 10 cm [5].

The diameter of this artery ranges from 1.5 mm [10] to more than 2 mm [3].

Venae comitantes are of similar caliber. The fourth perforating branch of the profunda femoris artery is also its end artery. It is usually small and pierces the adductor magnus muscle just proximal to the level of the hiatus of the adductor magnus. The vessel supplies muscular branches and may supply branches that ramify between the semimembranosus and semitendinosus muscles. Alternatively, the fourth perforating branch may supply a branch toward the subcutaneous tissue in the popliteal fossa, between the semimembranosus and biceps femoris muscles (Fig. 22.1).

C. Hou et al., *Surgical Atlas of Perforator Flaps: A Microsurgical Dissection Technique*,
DOI 10.1007/978-94-017-9834-1_22, © Springer Science+Business Media Dordrecht 2015

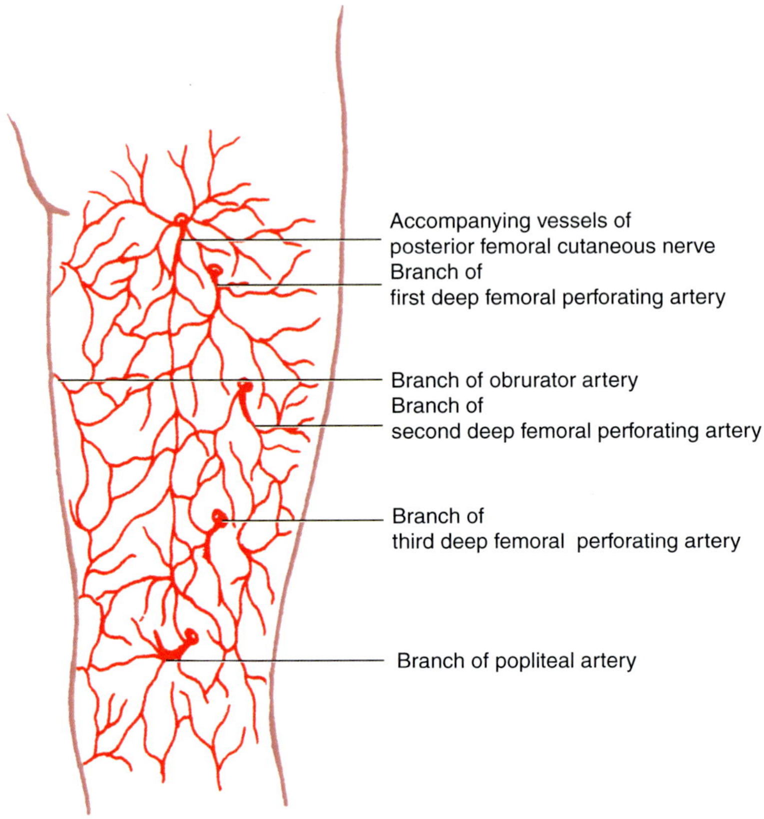

Fig. 22.1 Vascular anatomy of the posterior thigh perforator flap

22.2 Illustrative Case

A 47-year-old man presented popliteal fossa defect measuring 14 cm×6 cm after sustained traffic accident (Fig. 22.2).

Flap Design

The posterior branch of the third perforating artery (PFAP-3) emerges between the biceps femoris and semitendinosus muscles distally, about two-thirds of the distance from the ischial tuberosity and the midpoint between the medial and lateral tibial condyles. The line connecting these landmarks also marks the axis of the flap (Fig. 22.3).

The patient is placed in the prone or lateral position. A line is drawn from the ischium to the lateral femoral condyle.

Perforators from the profunda femoris artery are found on this line using a handheld Doppler probe or preoperatively using CT angiography (Fig. 22.4).

Flap Elevation

Dissection continues around the perforator with the most suitable size and position to obtain the desired pedicle length (Fig. 22.5).

The pedicle is followed to which it disappears behind the dense fibers of the linea aspera of the femur and the flap is ready for transfer (Fig. 22.6).

The flap was rotated 180° to cover the defect (Fig. 22.7).

The donor site was closed with a split-thickness skin graft (Fig. 22.8).

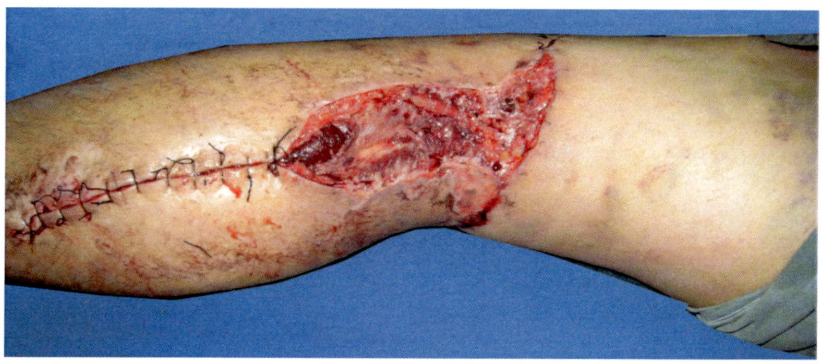

Fig. 22.2 Preoperative view

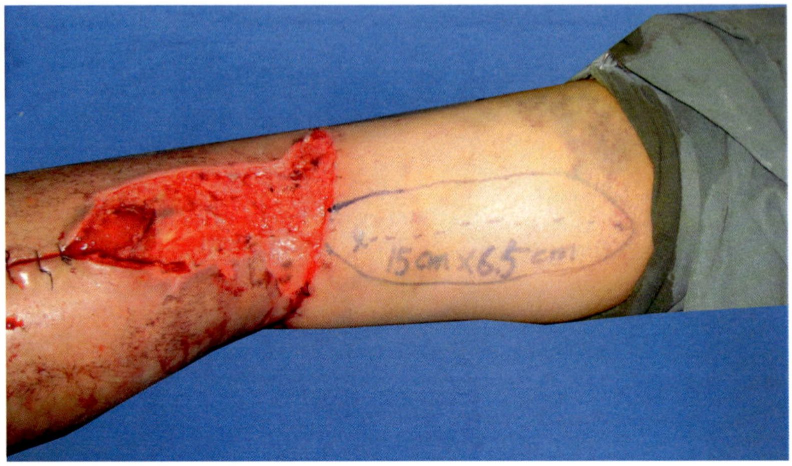

Fig. 22.3 Flap design

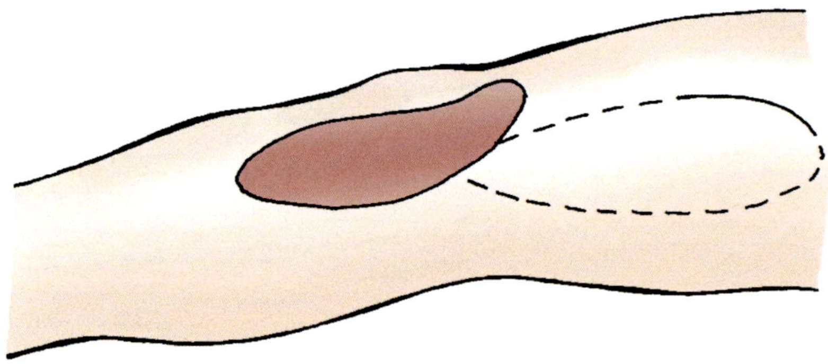

Fig. 22.4 Schematic drawing of the flap design

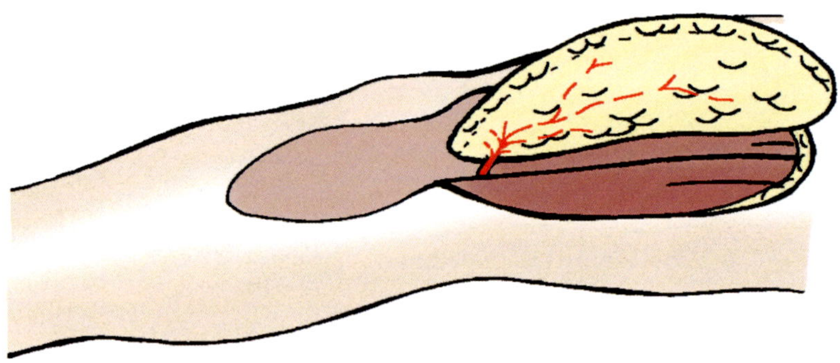

Fig. 22.5 Perforator vessel visualization

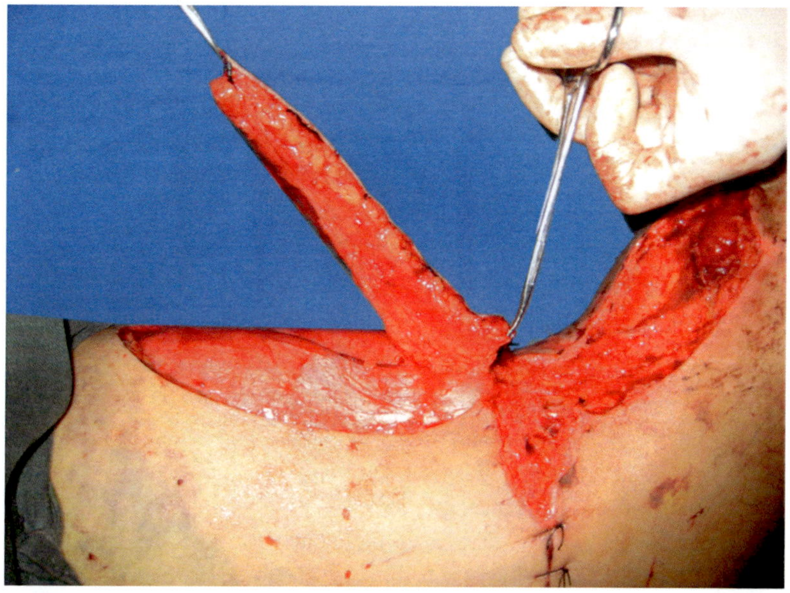

Fig. 22.6 Flap elevation

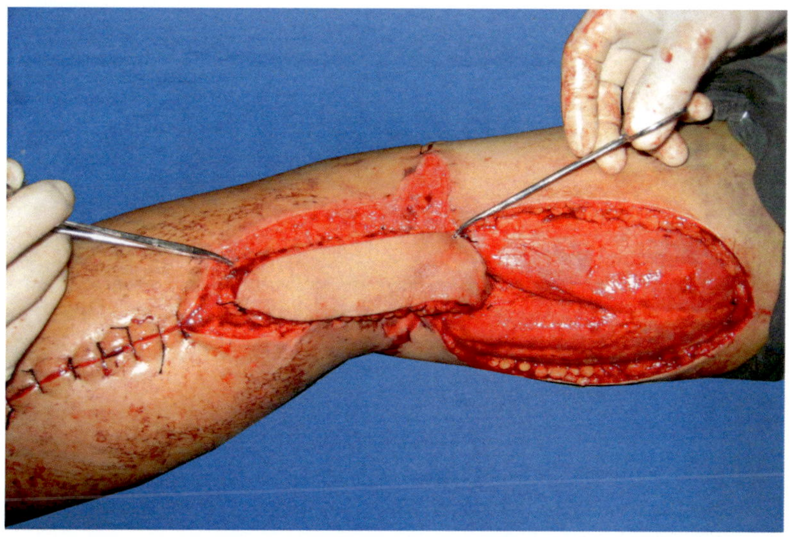

Fig. 22.7 Flap rotation

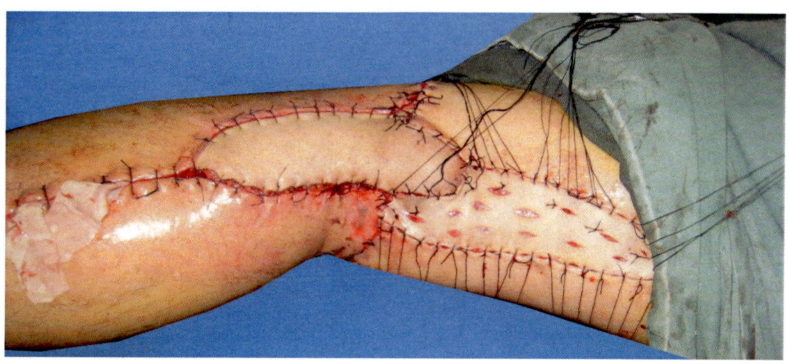

Fig. 22.8 Flap transfer and insetting

Pearls

The thickness of the flap, however, can be advantageous. The profunda femoris artery perforator (PFAP) flap has been used as a free flap for breast reconstruction [11].

The donor site less than 10 cm in width can usually be closed primarily.

Pitfalls

The vascular anatomy of the posterior thigh is highly variable, as it is with the entire thigh. Anatomical landmarks intended to specify the location of various cutaneous perforators can serve only as guidelines.

Audible Doppler examination is always essential to determine whether the perforators are present and to pinpoint their exact location.

The flap can be extremely thick. Secondary flap debulking may be necessary.

In males, the flap can be hirsute.

References

1. Hurwitz DJ. Closure of a large defect of the pelvic cavity by an extended compound myocutaneous flap based on the inferior gluteal artery. Br J Plast Surg. 1980;33(2):256–61.
2. Ramirez OM, Hurwitz DJ, Futrell JW. The expansive gluteus maximus flap. Plast Reconstr Surg. 1984; 74(6):757–70.
3. Song YG, Chen GZ, Song YL. The free thigh flap: a new free flap concept based on the septocutaneous artery. Br J Plast Surg. 1984;37(2):149–59.
4. Maruyama Y, Iwahira Y. Popliteo-posterior thigh fasciocutaneous island flap for closure around the knee. Br J Plast Surg. 1989;42(2):140–3; discussion 144–145.
5. Cormack GC, Lamberty BG. The blood supply of thigh skin. Plast Reconstr Surg. 1985;75(3):342–54.
6. Paletta C, Bartell T, Shehadi S. Applications of the posterior thigh flap. Ann Plast Surg. 1993;30(1): 41–7.
7. Lambert F, Cariou JL, Couturaud B, Bellavoir A. Fasciocutaneous flap of the posterior surface of the thigh with distal pedicle. Anatomical study and surgical value. A propos of 3 cases. Ann Chir Plast Esthet. 1996;41(2):145–54.
8. Ahmadzadeh R, Bergeron L, Tang M, Geddes CR, Morris SF. The posterior thigh perforator flap or profunda femoris artery perforator flap. Plast Reconstr Surg. 2007;119(1):194–200; discussion 201–192.
9. Rubin JA, Whetzel TP, Stevenson TR. The posterior thigh fasciocutaneous flap: vascular anatomy and clinical application. Plast Reconstr Surg. 1995;95(7): 1228–39.
10. Shimizu T, Fisher DR, Carmichael SW, Bite U. An anatomic comparison of septocutaneous free flaps from the thigh region. Ann Plast Surg. 1997;38(6): 604–10.
11. Allen RJ, Haddock NT, Ahn CY, Sadeghi A. Breast reconstruction with the profunda artery perforator flap. Plast Reconstr Surg. 2012;129(1):16e–23e.

Anterior Tibial Artery Perforator Flap

23

The anterior tibial artery perforator (ATAP) flap is vascularized by perforators of the anterior tibial artery and has been reported by several authors [1–6].

23.1 Vascular Anatomy

The anterior tibial (AT) artery begins at the inferior border of the popliteus muscle, branching from the bifurcation of the popliteal artery, passes between the two heads of the tibialis posterior, through the interosseous membrane, and to the deep part of the anterior leg. It then descends on the anterior surface of the interosseous membrane, moving closer to the tibia, and becomes the dorsalis pedis artery at the level of the ankle joint. The deep peroneal nerve accompanies the anterior tibial vessels. This is the source of motor branches to the anterior tibial muscle, which branch off from the main trunk within the proximal third of the lower leg (Fig. 23.1).

Several septocutaneous or musculocutaneous perforators originate from the anterior tibial artery [7, 8].

- The most proximal perforators of the anterior tibial artery are approximately 7 cm distal to the fibular head. The perforator then descends through the anterior intermuscular septum between the extensor digitorum longus and peroneus muscles and penetrates the deep fascia in the middle third of the lower leg.
- The middle septocutaneous or musculocutaneous perforators are derived from the anterior tibial artery approximately 12 cm distal to the tibial condyle. The perforators course downward through the intermuscular space between the anterior tibial muscle and the extensor digitorum longus muscle to penetrate the deep fascia at the junction of the upper and middle third of the lower leg.
- The most distal septocutaneous perforator arises from the anterior tibial system approximately 17–22 cm distal to the tibial condyle and runs caudally beneath the extensor digitorum longus muscle. The vessel courses anteriorly through the lateral intermuscular septum between the extensor digitorum and peroneus muscles or through the medial intermuscular septum between the anterior tibial muscle and the tibia. This perforator finally pierces the deep fascia to enter the skin of the lower two-thirds of the lower leg.

The dual venous system of the ATAP flap comprises the deep venae comitantes of the anterior tibial system or the superficial veins of the small saphenous system.

C. Hou et al., *Surgical Atlas of Perforator Flaps: A Microsurgical Dissection Technique*,
DOI 10.1007/978-94-017-9834-1_23, © Springer Science+Business Media Dordrecht 2015

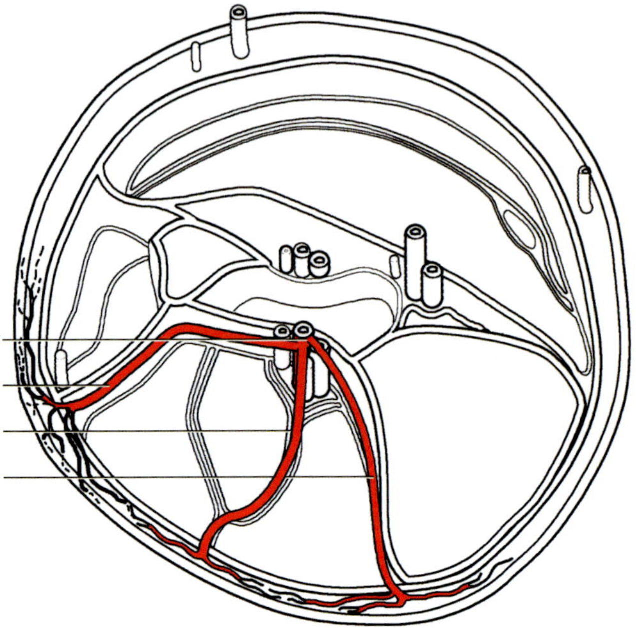

Fig. 23.1 Vascular anatomy of the anterior tibial artery

23.2 Illustrative Case

A 35-year-old woman sustained traffic accident. The resulting wound measured 8.5×5 cm over the anterior distal third of lower leg (Fig. 23.2).

Flap Design

Audible Doppler ultrasonography is very useful for locating perforators preoperatively (Fig. 23.3).

The flap is outlined on the anterolateral aspect of the middle third of the lower leg, incorporating at least one perforator.

Flap Elevation

An incision is made along the anterior edge of the marked flap. The lateral border of the flap was raised first until the anterior tibial perforators are exposed.

The perforators are dissected back to the deep anterior tibial vessels. Several perforators are typically found in the distal third of the lower leg. The medial incision can then be completed and the whole flap elevated suprafascially. An island ATAP flap with a single perforator allows unimpeded transfer as a local flap to an adjacent defect (Fig. 23.4).

Flap Transfer

The flap was then rotated 150° to reach the recipient site (Fig. 23.5).

Follow-Up

The flap showed good texture and contour matches postoperatively (Fig. 23.6).

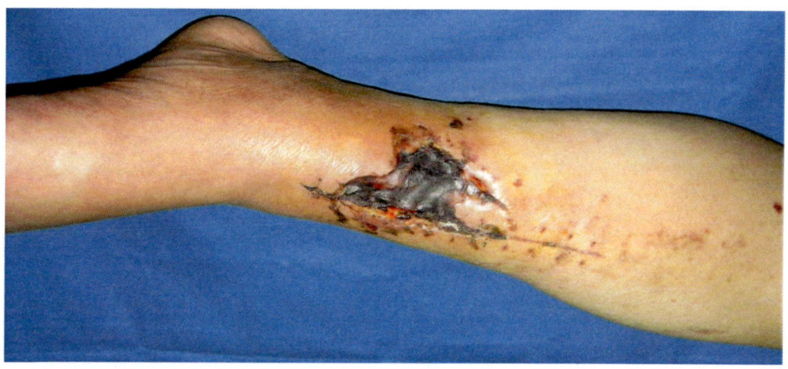

Fig. 23.2 Preoperative view

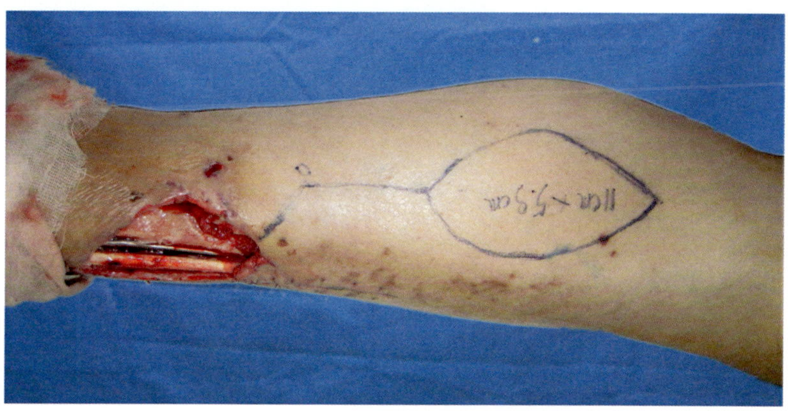

Fig. 23.3 Flap design

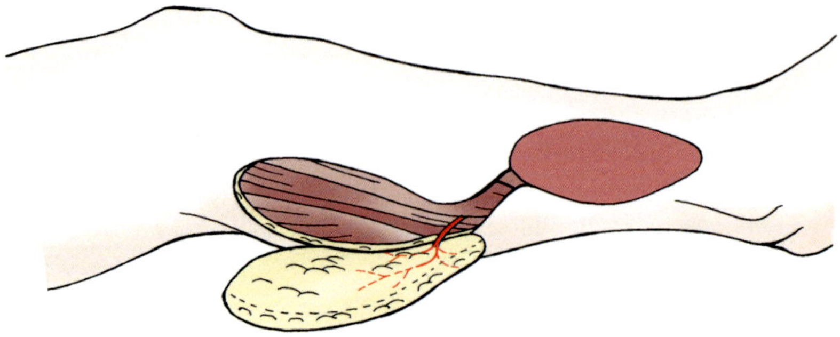

Fig. 23.4 Schematic drawing of the flap design

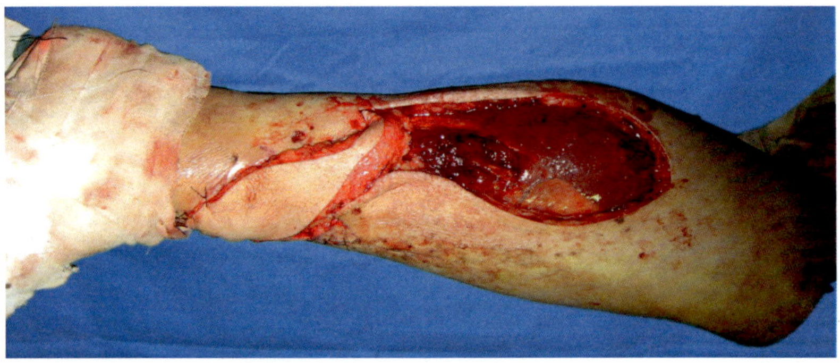

Fig. 23.5 Flap rotation

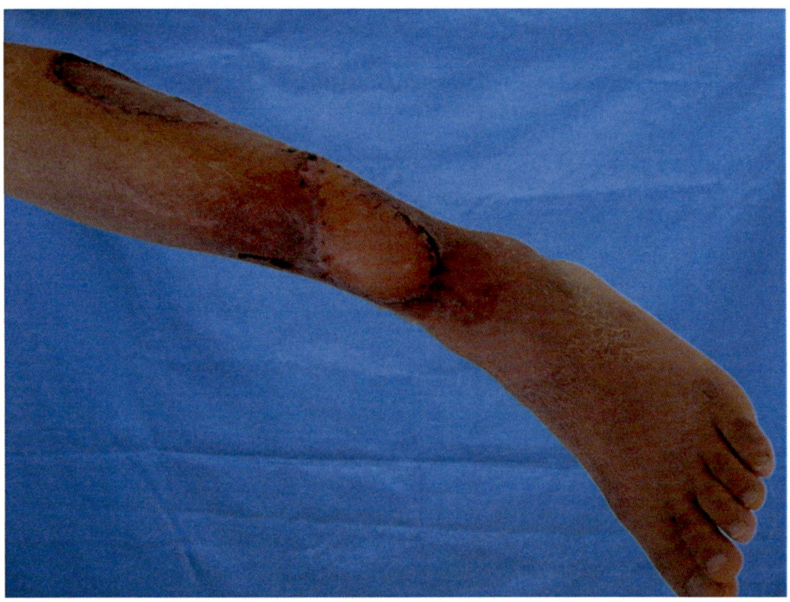

Fig. 23.6 Follow-up

Pearls

Due to sufficient blood supply of the flaps, there was no distinct restriction on the length-to-width ratio.

The flap produced a good contour.

The thin consistency of the flap allowed patients to wear normal shoes once healing was complete.

Pitfalls

The number and location of anterior tibial artery perforators can be variable or even absent.

During flap inset, undue tension on or twisting of the vessels will compromise circulation and therefore flap survival [9].

References

1. Kim NG, Lee KS, Choi TH, et al. Aesthetic reconstruction of lower leg defects using a new anterolateral lower leg perforator flap. J Plast Reconstr Aesthet Surgery JPRAS. 2008;61(8):934–8.
2. Morrison WA, Shen TY. Anterior tibial artery flap: anatomy and case report. Br J Plast Surg. 1987; 40(3):230–5.
3. Torii S, Namiki Y, Hayashi Y. Anterolateral leg island flap. Br J Plast Surg. 1987;40(3):236–40.
4. Kilinc H, Bilen BT, Arslan A. A novel flap to repair medial and lateral malleolar defects: anterior tibial artery perforator-based adipofascial flap. Ann Plast Surg. 2006;57(4):396–401.
5. Rad AN, Christy MR, Rodriguez ED, Brazio P, Rosson GD. The anterior tibialis artery perforator (ATAP) flap for traumatic knee and patella defects: clinical cases and anatomic study. Ann Plast Surg. 2010;64(2):210–6.
6. Xu Z, Chenglin L, Zhiwen N, Sumin W, Ruxia Y, Xu M. Use of flap based on anterior tibial artery for free transfer. J Reconstr Microsurg. 2008;24(2): 103–10.
7. Panagiotopoulos K, Soucacos PN, Korres DS, et al. Anatomical study and colour Doppler assessment of the skin perforators of the anterior tibial artery and possible clinical applications. J Plast Reconstr Aesthet Surg JPRAS. 2009;62(11):1524–9.
8. Schaverien M, Saint-Cyr M. Perforators of the lower leg: analysis of perforator locations and clinical application for pedicled perforator flaps. Plast Reconstr Surg. 2008;122(1):161–70.
9. Wang RL, Li N, Jiang CH, Guo F, Su T. Anterior tibial artery perforator flap for reconstruction of intraoral defects. J Oral Maxillofac Surg Off J Am Assoc Oral Maxillofac Surg. 2014;72(4):804–10.

24 Posterior Tibial Artery Perforator Flap

A skin flap from the medial leg based on the posterior tibial artery and its cutaneous branches was first described by Zhang and colleagues in 1983 [1].

24.1 Vascular Anatomy

The posterior tibial artery is almost always present and is normally the largest terminal branch of the popliteal artery or tibioperoneal trunk [2].

As it reaches the ankle, the posterior tibial artery lies between the flexor digitorum longus and soleus muscles and Achilles tendon to almost assume a somewhat subcutaneous path [3].

Cutaneous perforators arise from the posterior tibial artery at unpredictable intervals (Fig. 24.1).

There are three distinct clusters of perforators for the posterior tibial artery at the following distances proximal to the medial malleolus: (1) 4–9 cm, (2) 13–18 cm, and (3) 21–26 cm.

Perforators with the largest caliber were typically present in the proximal two-thirds of the leg (Fig. 24.2).

24.2 Case 1: Distally Based Perforator Propeller Flap for Plate Exposure

A 60-year-old female suffered from an open Pilon fracture (Fig. 24.3). The skin over the medial malleolar area was necrotic after plate fixation, although MIPPO technique was applied (Fig. 24.4).

After debridement, the defect was measured 4 × 5 cm with plate exposure. We designed a posterior tibial artery perforator flap to cover the wound (Fig. 24.5).

A 7 cm long explore incision was made along the Achilles tendon down to the deep fascia. The fasciocutaneous was anchored with each other by some stitches to avoid separation. Then the deep fascia was elevated anteriorly to find perforators issuing from the deep posterior tibial artery. The perforator was identified at 9 cm above the medial malleolus. The vascular bundle was one perforating artery (arrow) with diameter of 1.0 mm accompanied by two veins (Fig. 24.6). The width of the vascular bundle was 1.5 cm with 3 cm in length.

The designed flap was remeasured and adjusted (Fig. 24.7). The big flap blade was 10 × 4 cm; the small flap blade was 4 × 2 cm (Fig. 24.8).

The flap was propelled to the recipient site in clockwise, with good circulation (Fig. 24.9).

In postoperative day 2, the distal third of the flap showed venous congestion and swelling and finally tension blister occurred. Multiple small incisions were made over the flap to let venous blood out and finally circulation recovered. The reason for venous congestion in this case may be the smaller size of the flap. After insetting, skin tension was developed due to stretching by suture (Fig. 24.10).

The flap was eventually survived, with minor distal superficial necrosis, which healed without further management (Fig. 24.11).

C. Hou et al., *Surgical Atlas of Perforator Flaps: A Microsurgical Dissection Technique*,
DOI 10.1007/978-94-017-9834-1_24, © Springer Science+Business Media Dordrecht 2015

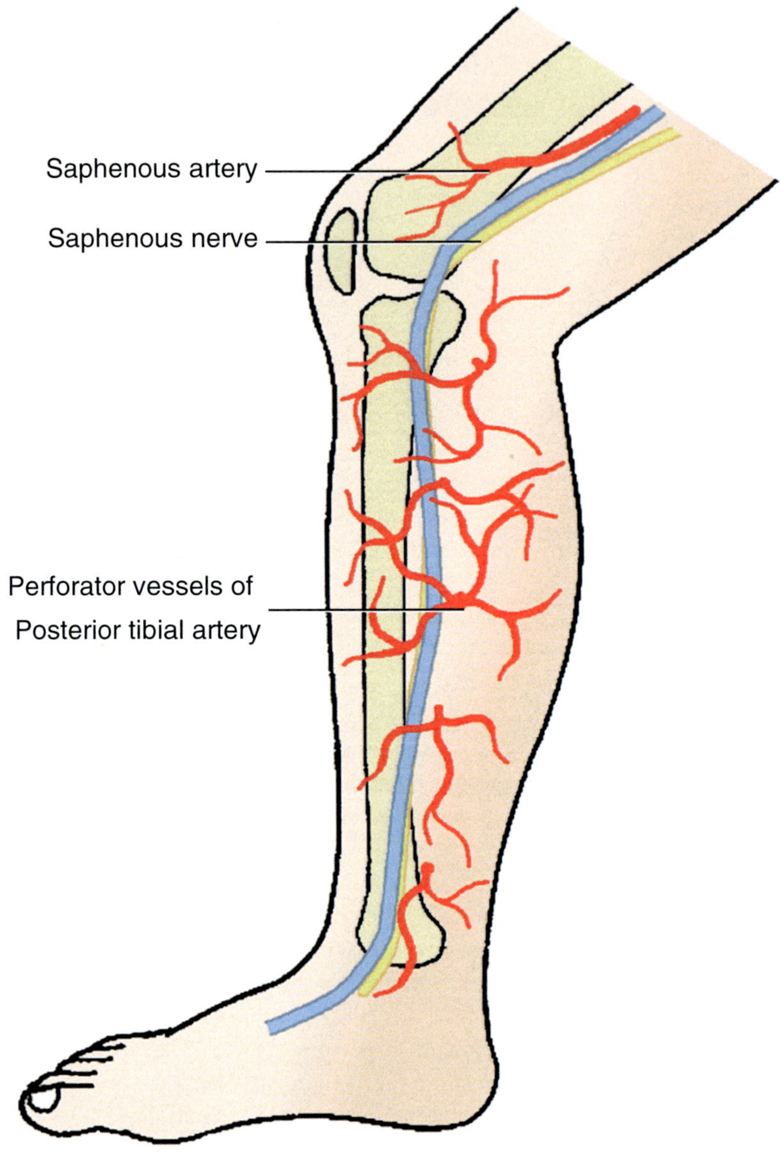

Fig. 24.1 Vascular anatomy of the posterior tibial artery

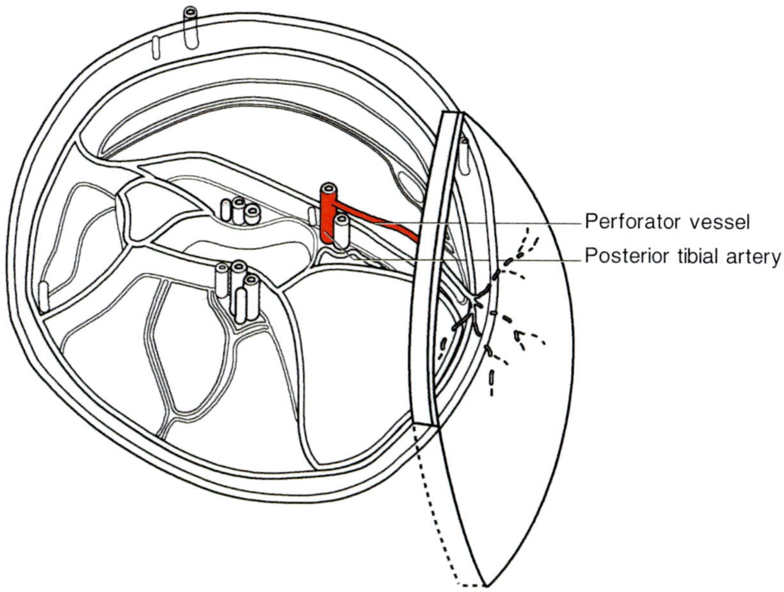

Fig. 24.2 The perforators of the posterior tibial artery

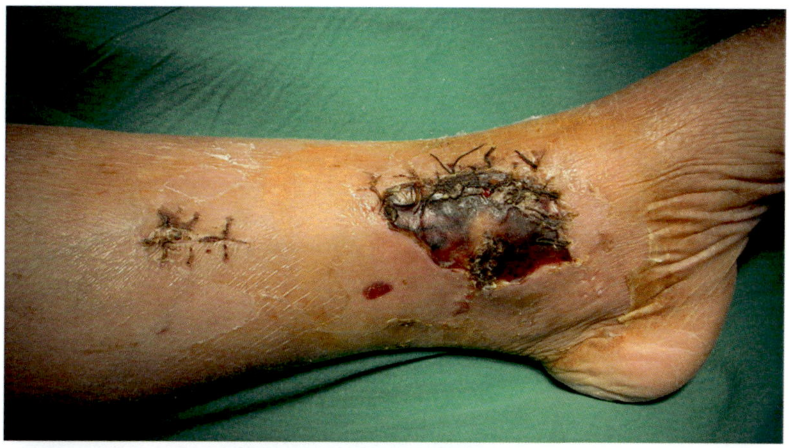

Fig. 24.3 Preoperative view

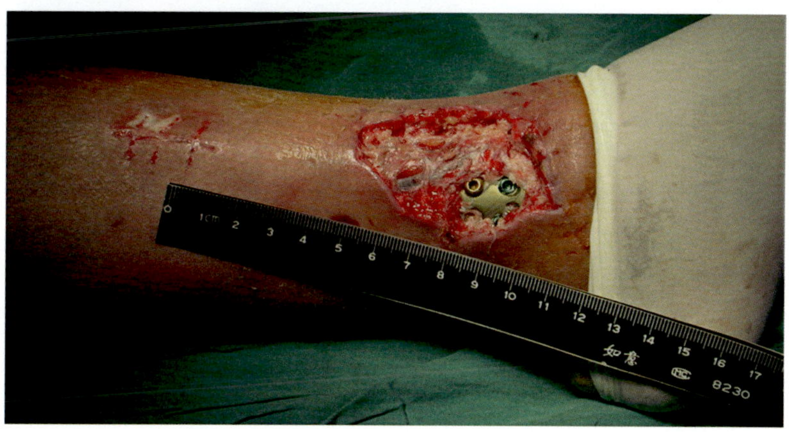

Fig. 24.4 The wound after thorough debridement

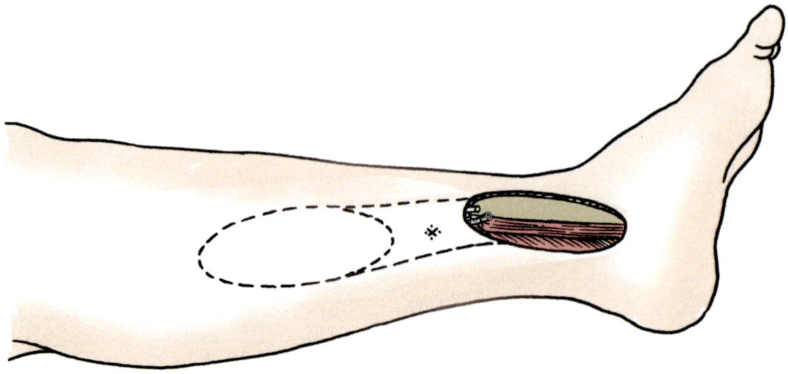

Fig. 24.5 Schematic drawing of the flap design

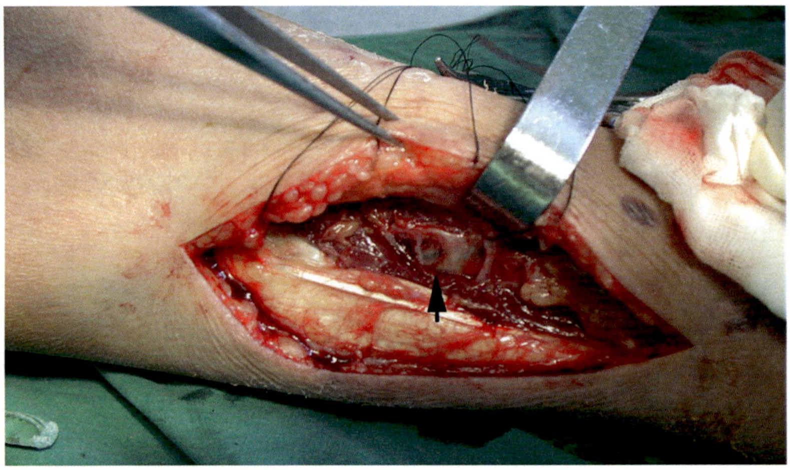

Fig. 24.6 Perforator vessel visualization

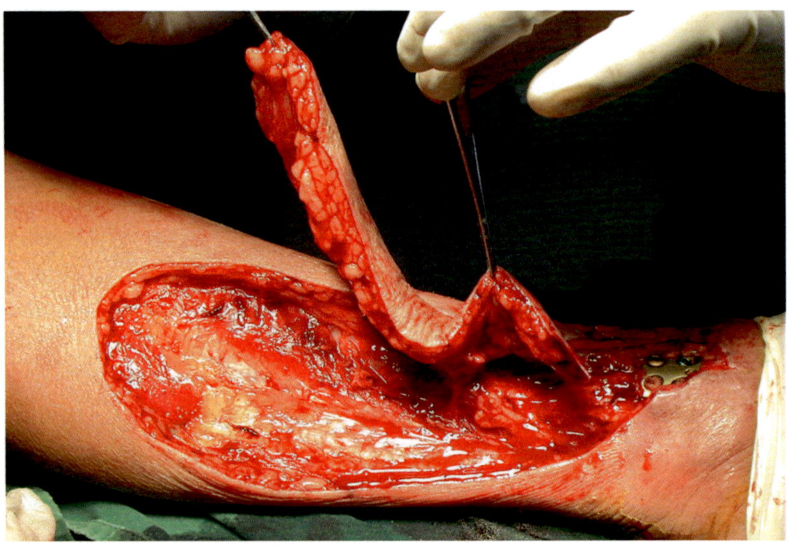

Fig. 24.7 Flap elevation

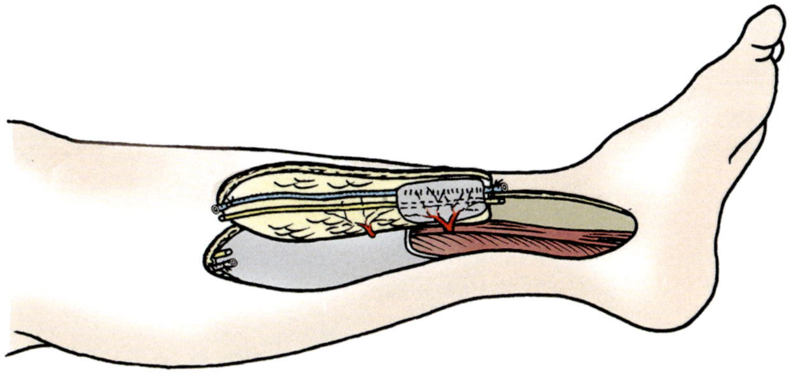

Fig. 24.8 Schematic drawing of the flap elevation

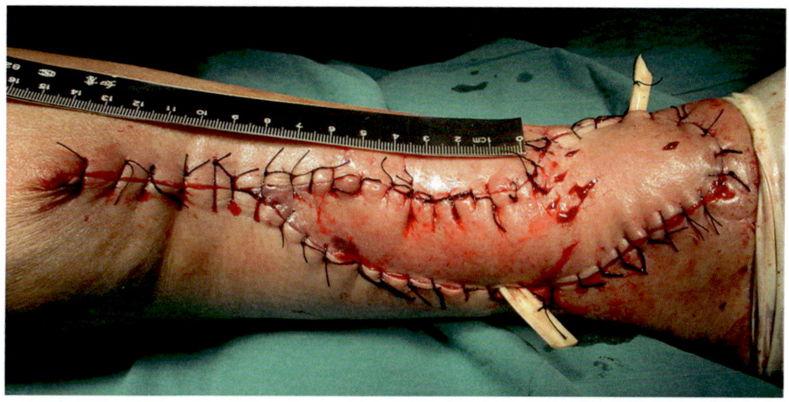

Fig. 24.9 Flap transfer and insetting

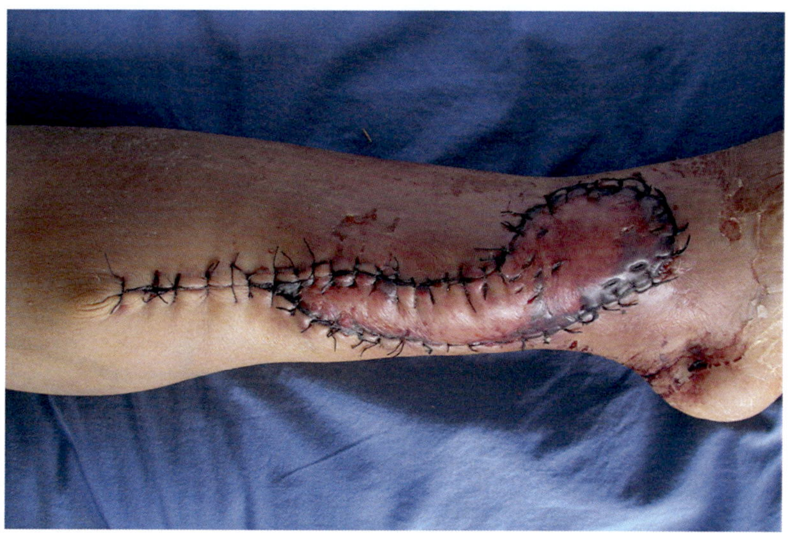

Fig. 24.10 Postoperative view

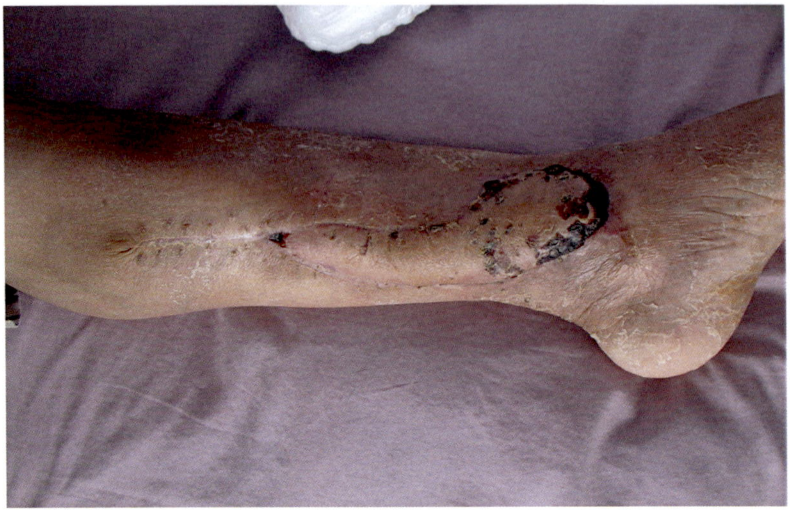

Fig. 24.11 Follow-up

24.3 Case 2: Distally Perforator-Plus Flap for Achilles Coverage

A 12-year-old boy injured his right heel in a bicycle spoke, resulting in Achilles rupture and overlying skin avulsion. After primary suture, he was referred to us 2 weeks later because of infection and skin necrosis. After thorough debridement, the skin defect measured 5×4 cm with ruptured Achilles tendon exposure (Fig. 24.12).

The tendon was repaired to calcaneus by two suture anchors. A distally based posterior tibial artery perforator-adipofascial-pedicled flap was designed to cover the heel defect. The closest perforator located 6 cm above the medial malleolar tip (a septal perforator). The flap was raised in propeller shape, with a proximal large fasciocutaneous blade of 4×10 cm and a distal small cutaneous blade of 3×3 cm (Fig. 24.13).

The fasciocutaneous flap was rotated 180° in clockwise to reach the posterior heel defect with no tension. The thin cutaneous flap was rotated proximally to cover the pedicle. The donor site was closed in tension-release suture and skin graft. Postoperatively, the flap demonstrated a grade 2 swelling. However, the flap survived uneventfully (Fig. 24.14).

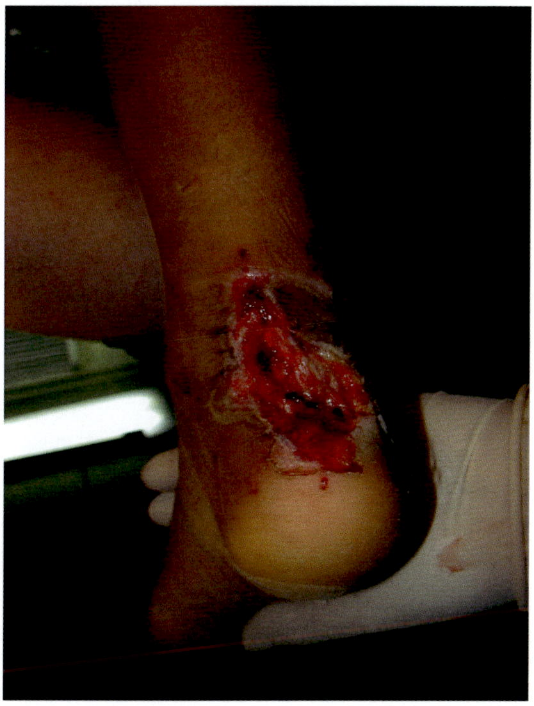

Fig. 24.12 Preoperative view

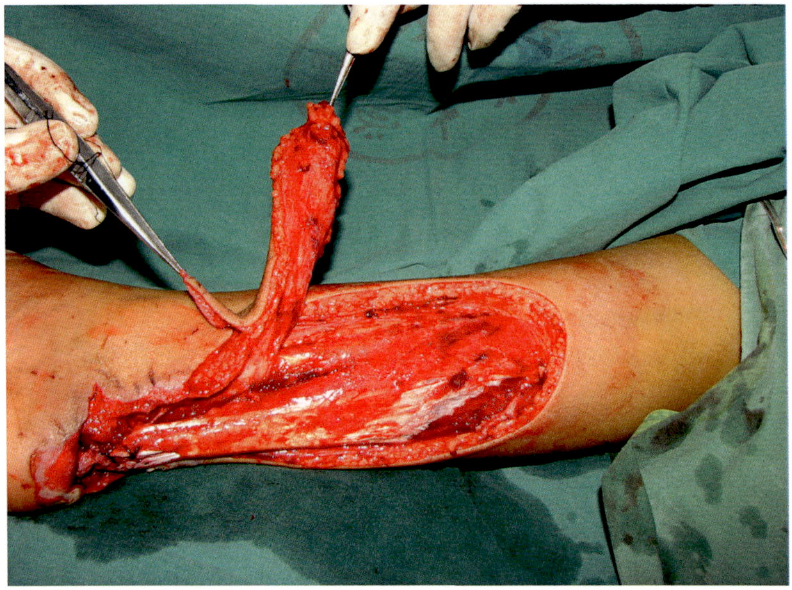

Fig. 24.13 Flap elevation

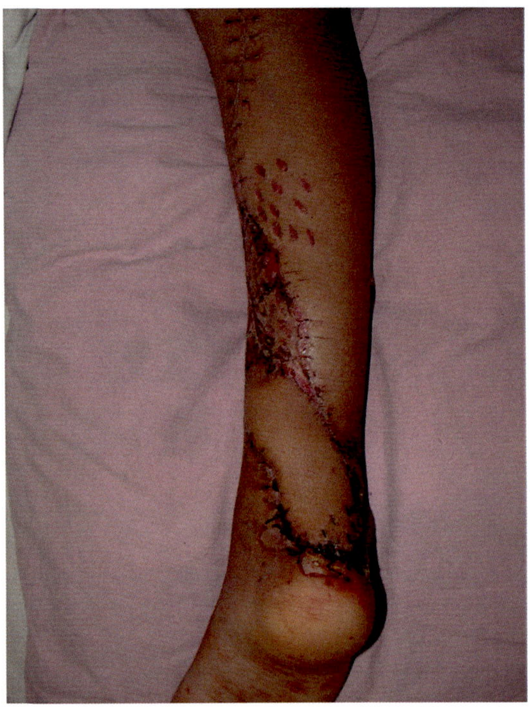

Fig. 24.14 Postoperative view

Pearls

Except in the most obese patients, a thin flap is available if using a skin territory based on more distal perforators.

A portion of the saphenous nerve that accompanies the great saphenous vein can be taken with the flap to allow reinnervation.

Care must be taken not to close the deep fascia tightly or at all to avoid iatrogenic compartment syndrome. A small fascial defect can result in muscle herniation, and opening the deep fascia widely or leaving it open may always be preferable.

Pitfalls

Congenital absence of the posterior tibial artery is rare, but atherosclerotic peripheral vascular disease with occlusion is not. Inflow to the lower limb must be assessed before selecting the donor site.

Posterior tibial perforators are consistently grouped in each third of the leg [4], but are unpredictable individually.

The multi-detector-row CT and Doppler helps precisely locate the essential perforator, and approaching this flap as a free-style local or free flap will be necessary.

References

1. Zhang SC. [Clinical application of medial skin flap of leg–analysis of 9 cases]. Zhonghua wai ke za zhi [Chin J Surg]. 1983;21(12):743–5.
2. Tang M, Mao Y, Almutairi K, Morris SF. Three-dimensional analysis of perforators of the posterior leg. Plast Reconstr Surg. 2009;123(6):1729–38.
3. Carriquiry C, Aparecida Costa M, Vasconez LO. An anatomic study of the septocutaneous vessels of the leg. Plast Reconstr Surg. 1985;76(3):354–63.
4. Schaverien M, Saint-Cyr M. Perforators of the lower leg: analysis of perforator locations and clinical application for pedicled perforator flaps. Plast Reconstr Surg. 2008;122(1):161–70.

25 Peroneal Artery Perforator Flap

In 1983, Donski and Fogdestam first described a distally perforator-based sural fasciocutaneous flap for heel coverage. The flap was based on perforating branches from the posterolateral septum issued from the peroneal artery at 5–7 cm above the lateral malleolus.

On the basis of the results of their preliminary cadaver dissection and their clinical experience, Aoki et al. [1] proved that the vascular anastomosis between the superficial sural artery and the septocutaneous perforator of the peroneal artery forms an arterial network around the entire length of the distal sural nerve.

The clinical and anatomical findings suggested that the sural nerve can be preserved to prevent surgically induced paresthesia [2].

25.1 Vascular Anatomy

Briefly, the superficial sural artery from the popliteal, the septocutaneous perforators from posterior tibial (medial side) and peroneal artery (lateral side), and the myocutaneous perforators from gastrocnemius and soleus form a three dimensional vascular architecture of the posterior lower leg integument. There are prominent longitudinal orientation or axiality of the circulation of fascial, paraneural (sural nerve), and perivenous (lesser saphenous vein) vascular plexuses. There are 4–5 axial communications between this longitudinal neuro-veno-adipofascial plexus and the posterolateral septocutaneous perforators issued from the peroneal artery. The lowest anastomosis from the peroneal artery, the posterolateral supramalleolar perforator, usually 1.2 mm in origin diameter, was located approximately 5 cm above the lateral malleolus. With a distal axial perforator perfusion, blood can run a long distance along the lower resistance longitudinal vascular plexuses and result in a large flap survival without arterial ischemia (Fig. 25.1).

There are two venous systems in the calf and sural region, i.e., superficial venous system in the subcutaneous adipose tissue and deep venous system accompanied to the main artery (venae comitantes). Both of these vessels are provided with valves to direct venous return proximally. The superficial and deep venous systems are connected with each other by perforating and communicating veins through the deep fascia.

As a distally based sural neuro-veno-fasciocutaneous flap was raised, all the proximal vessels are cut and ligated, so only the distal vessels have functions for flap circulation. Drainage of venous blood of the flap was thought in the same way as arterial perfusion. It was drained first by the avalvular small venous plexuses of fascial, paraneural, and perivenous to the distal perforating or communicating veins and then to the deep venous system and returned in orthograde direction. Large subcutaneous lesser saphenous vein has no functional role for venous return in distally based sural flaps.

C. Hou et al., *Surgical Atlas of Perforator Flaps: A Microsurgical Dissection Technique*,
DOI 10.1007/978-94-017-9834-1_25,

25.2 Case 1: Flap Based on the Distal Most Septocutaneous Perforator

A 56-year-old man sustained a traffic accident injury on his left ankle over the lateral malleolus, resulting a wound measured 10 × 6 cm (Fig. 25.2).

Flap Design

After debridement, a 12 × 7 cm peroneal artery perforator flap supplied by a pivot point 6 cm above the lateral malleolus was designed in an eccentric propeller shape (Fig. 25.3). The longitudinal axis of the flap was a line from the mid-popliteal point to the midpoint between the Achilles tendon and lateral malleolus (Fig. 25.4).

Flap Elevation

An incision was made along the anterior border of the flap. The terminal peroneal septocutaneous perforating vessel was located in the fascial plexus of the flap by careful dissection. During the dissection procedure, particular attention was paid to preserve the vascular pedicle (Fig. 25.5).

The lesser saphenous vein and sural nerve traveled through the proposed flap; they were dissected out and left intact (Fig. 25.6). Dissection of both the vein and nerve was carried out under loupe magnification; the accompanying vessels were divided meticulously from the lesser saphenous vein and sural nerve and included in the flap. The flap was completely elevated and was attached to the donor site only with the perforating vessels (Fig. 25.7).

With only the terminal peroneal perforating branch as the pedicle, the flap was raised in an island form above the deep fascia. Loose perivascular tissue around the perforating vessels was cautiously removed to reduce the likelihood of strangulation of the perforator during flap rotation. Perfusion was checked before flap rotation by waiting for a few minutes (Fig. 25.8).

Flap Transfer

The flap was then rotated 120° to reach the recipient site. The long blade filled the defect without tension; the minor skin paddle was used to help close a large part of the donor site (Fig. 25.9).

Flap Insetting

Flap transfer and split-thickness skin graft of the donor site is shown in Fig. 25.10.

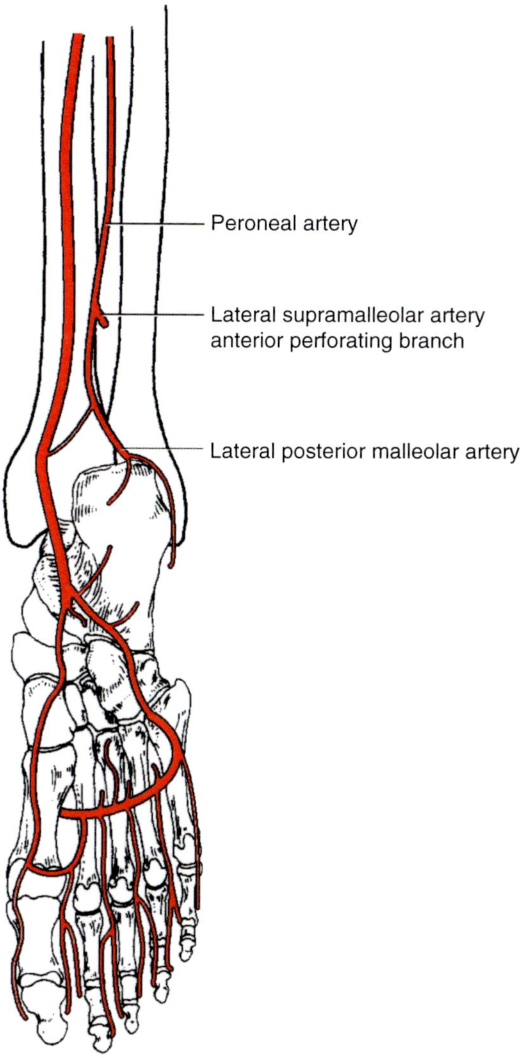

Fig. 25.1 Vascular anatomy of the peroneal artery

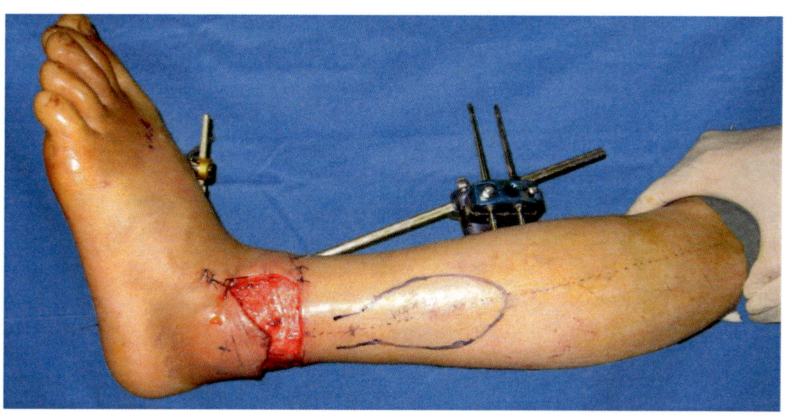

Fig. 25.2 Preoperative view and the flap design

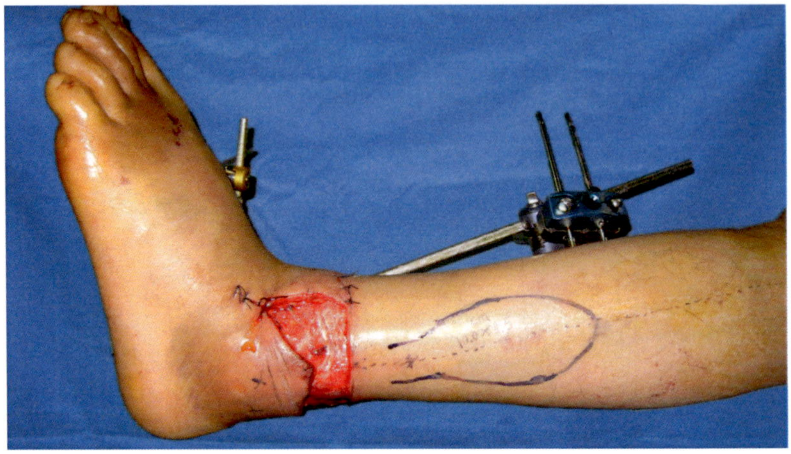

Fig. 25.3 Flap design

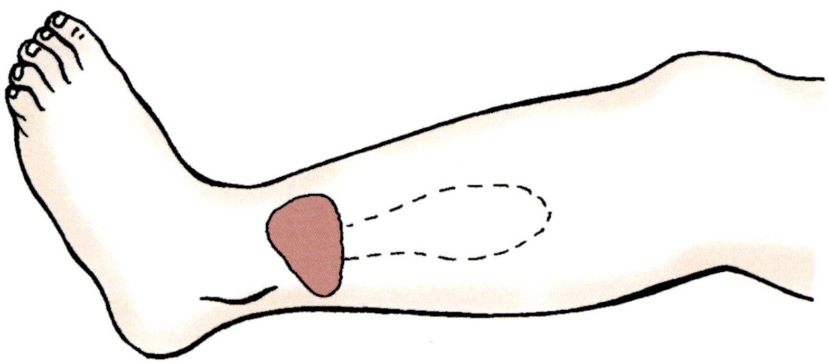

Fig. 25.4 Schematic drawing of the flap design

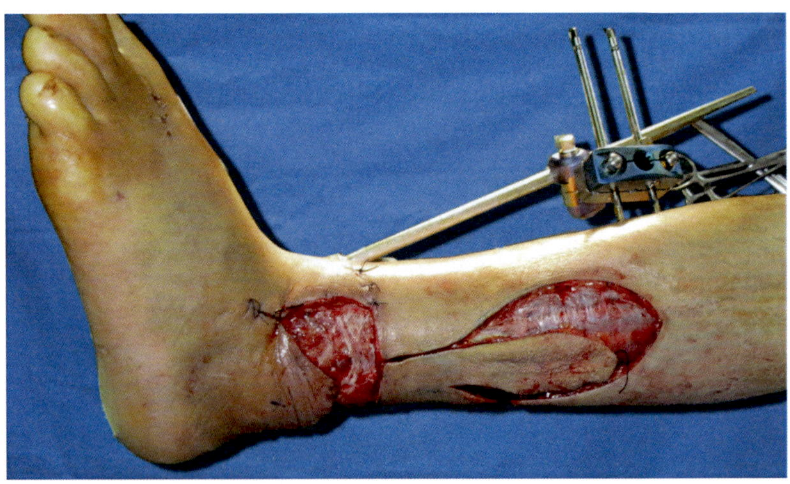

Fig. 25.5 Perforator vessel visualization

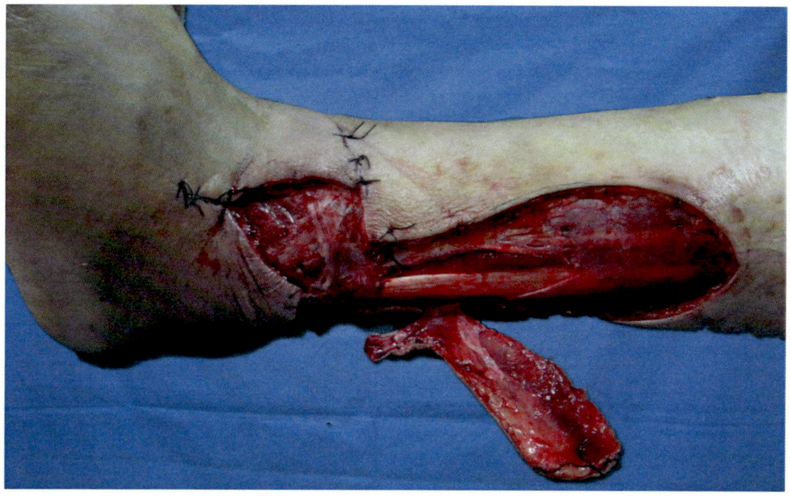

Fig. 25.6 Flap elevation

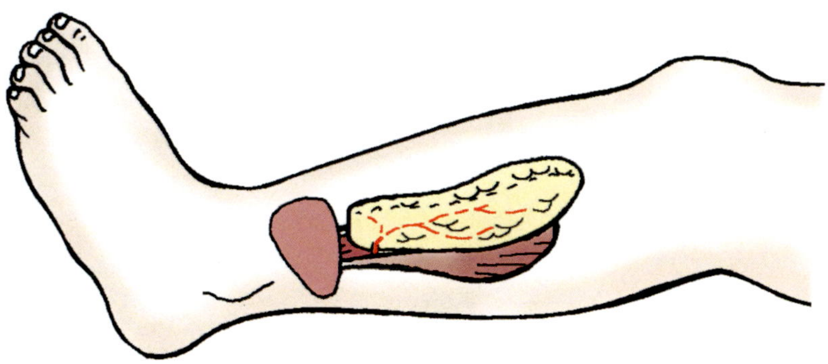

Fig. 25.7 Schematic drawing of the flap elevation

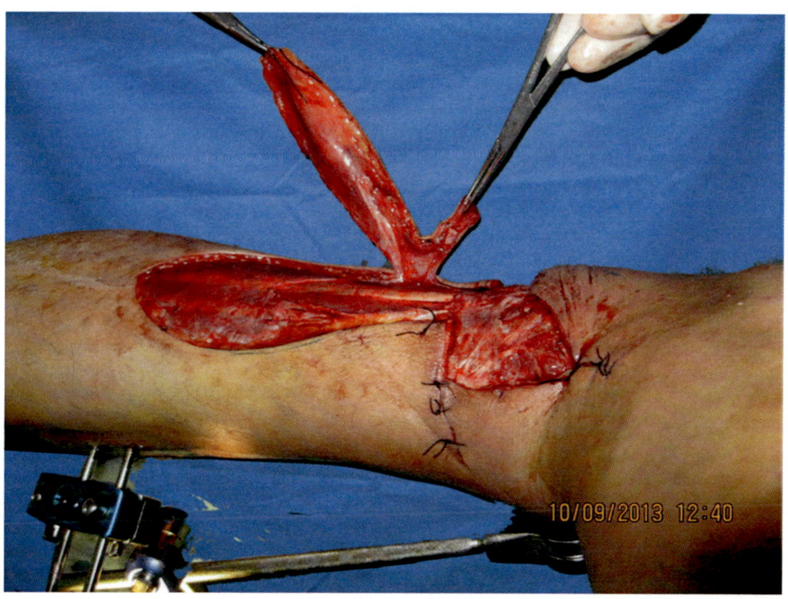

Fig. 25.8 Flap rotation

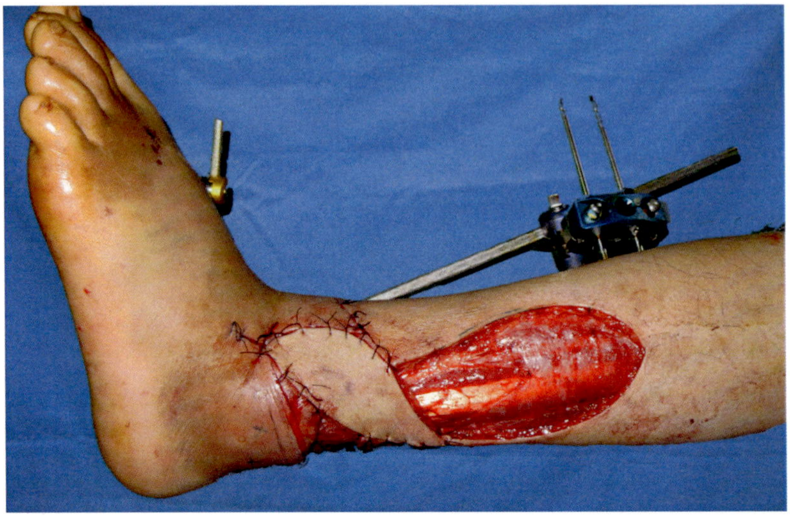

Fig. 25.9 Flap transfer

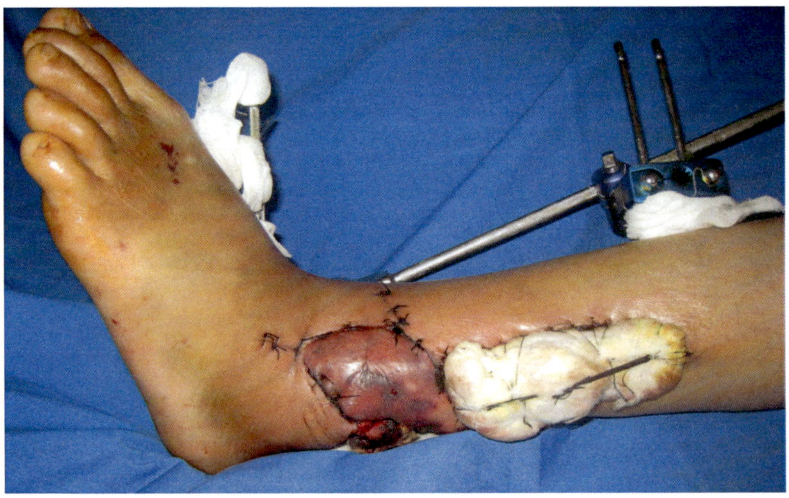

Fig. 25.10 Flap insetting

25.3 Case 2: Distally Fasciomyocutaneous Flap Based on the Distal Most Septocutaneous Perforator

A 42-year-old mine worker was referred to us after calcaneal comminuted fracture and skin defect of his heel for 4 months. The shape of the calcaneus, though malunited, was acceptable. The skin defect was 11 × 8 cm, with no heel pad remaining.

A distally based peroneal artery perforator-pedicled sural fasciomyocutaneous flap was designed to cover the heel defect (Fig. 25.11). The fasciocutaneous flap measured 12 × 9 cm, and the attached lateral gastrocnemius muscle flap measured 7 × 5 cm. The thin muscle flap (1–1.5 cm thickness) was used to cover the plantar heel to provide a pad for weight bearing (Fig. 25.12). The proximal sural nerve was harvested for extra 3 cm and coapted to the calcaneal branch of tibial nerve in an end-to-side fashion (Fig. 25.13).

Although venous congestion occurred after operation, no tension blister appeared. The flap survived completely and the wound healed eventually (Fig. 25.14).

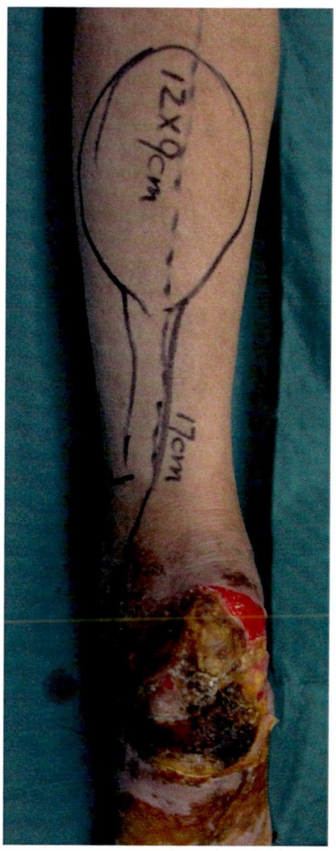

Fig. 25.11 Preoperative view and the flap design

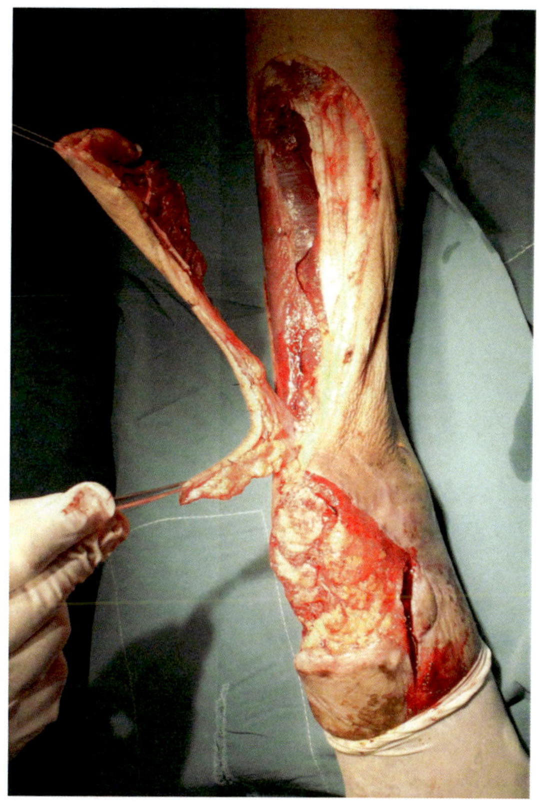

Fig. 25.12 Flap elevation

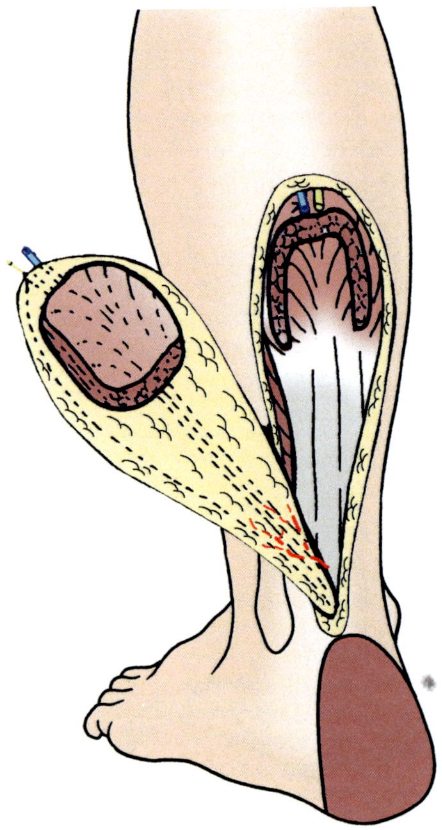

Fig. 25.13 Schematic drawing of the flap elevation

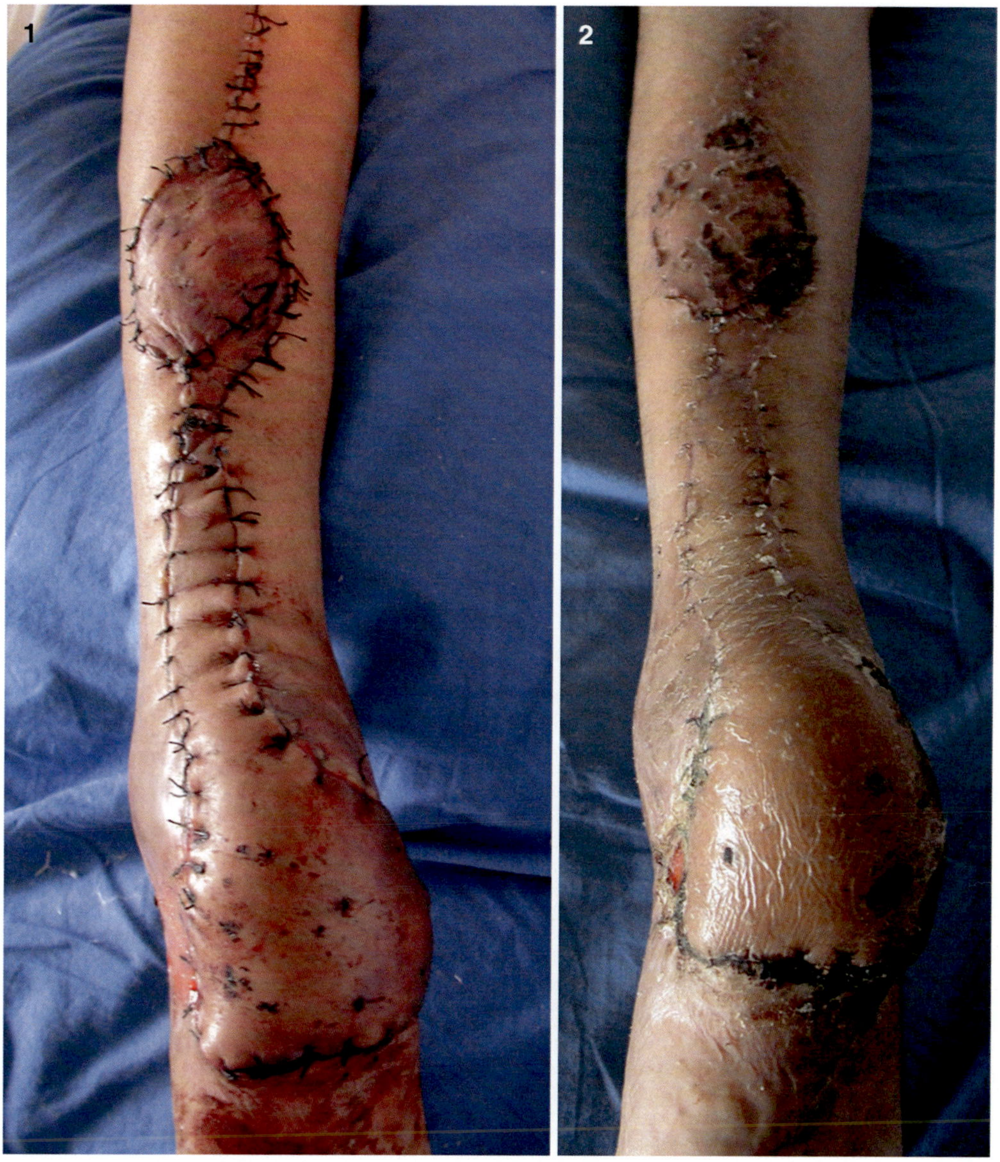

Fig. 25.14 Postoperative view

25.4 Case 3: Distally Based Sural Fasciomyocutaneous Flap with Perforator-Plus Adipofascial Pedicle

A 53-year-old man was referred to our department for an iatrogenic wound infection for 3 weeks after plate fixation for distal tibia fracture of his left leg (Fig. 25.15). The anterior tibialis tendon and metal plate was exposed. Bacteria culture showed a combined infection of *Staphylococcus aureus* and *Escherichia coli*. After preoperative intravenous antibiotic therapy for 1 week, the patient underwent debridement and flap coverage in one stage. The skin defect was 7×5 cm in size. The dead space measured by filling of saline water during operation was 56 ml.

Distally based sural fasciomyocutaneous flap was designed for coverage of the skin defect and filling of the dead space with high metabolic muscle flap to cure the infection. The fasciocutaneous flap was measured 8×5 cm in size with an adipofascial pedicle of 7 cm long and 3 cm wide with 1 cm skin bridge (Fig. 25.16). The attached muscle flap was 4×3 cm in size and 2 cm in thickness. After the flap elevation and pneumatic tourniquet removal, the flap showed good vascularization as blood oozing from the gastrocnemius muscle fragment was observed in 2 min (Fig. 25.17).

The lesser saphenous vein was ligated from the distal pedicle to prevent venous engorgement of the foot, thus reducing the venous load for reverse return of flap (Fig. 25.18).

The flap was open transferred with no tension or compression. The muscle was inserted beneath the anterior tibialis tendon to fill the dead space, and the fasciocutaneous flap was inset to the overlying skin defect. The flap survived completely with no complication (Fig. 25.19).

The patients was followed up for 18 months; no weakness in heel-lifting force was observed (Fig. 25.20).

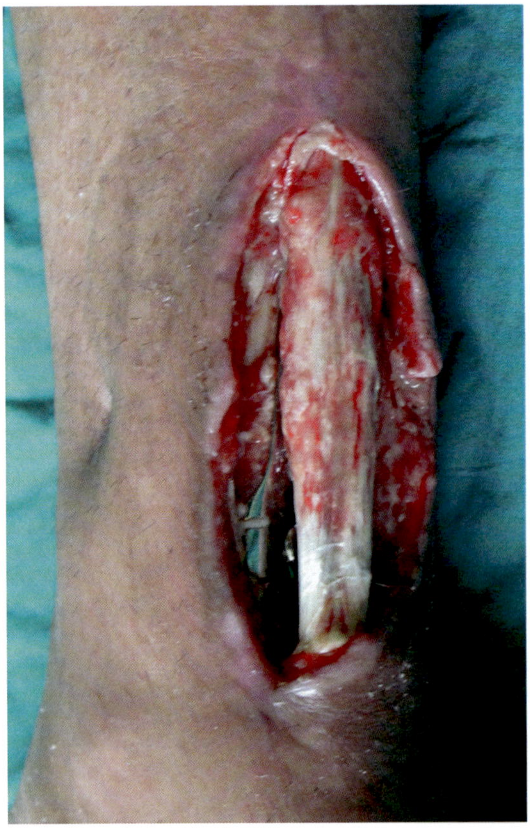

Fig. 25.15 Preoperative view

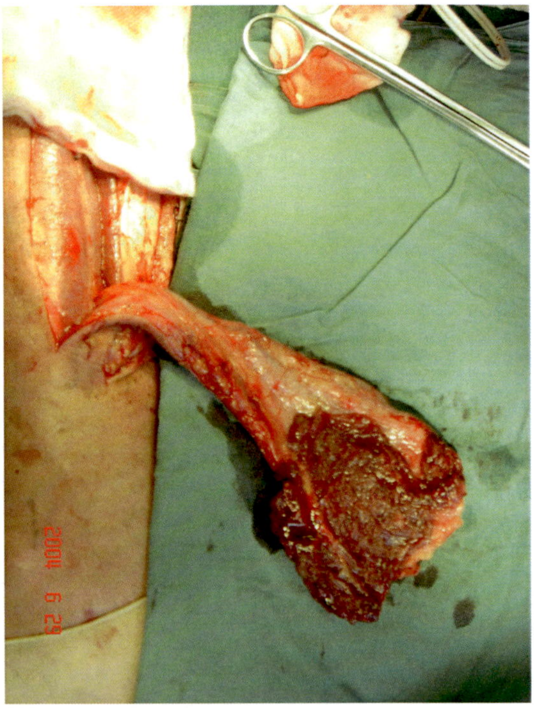

Fig. 25.16 Flap elevation

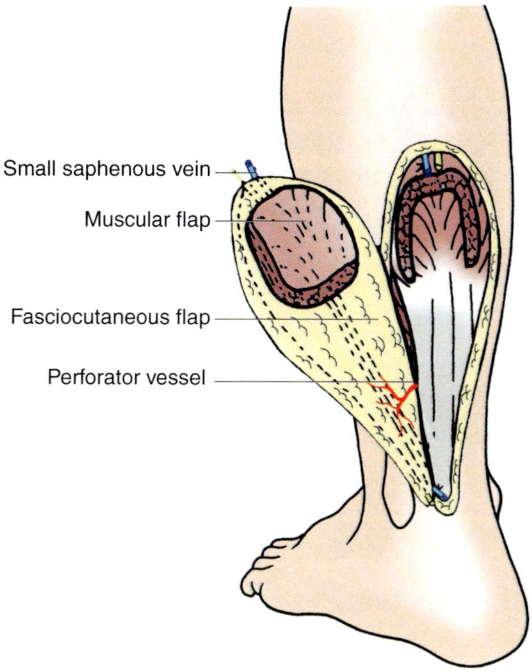

Fig. 25.17 Schematic drawing of the flap elevation

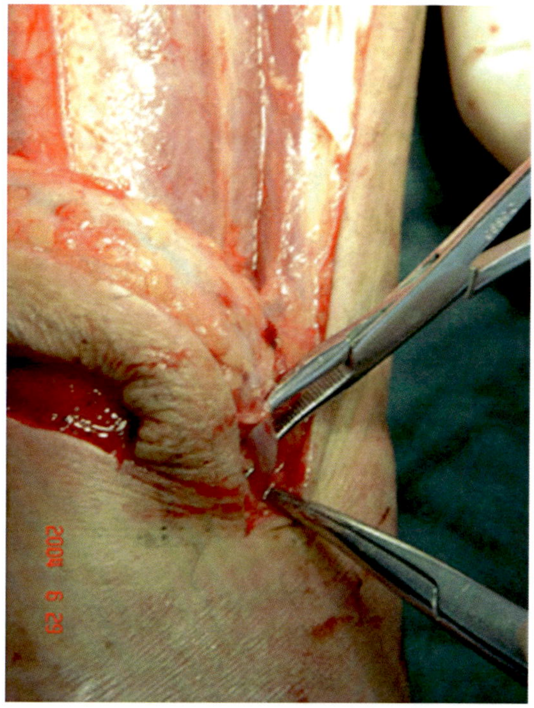

Fig. 25.18 Ligation of the distal ingress lesser saphenous vein to prevent venous congestion

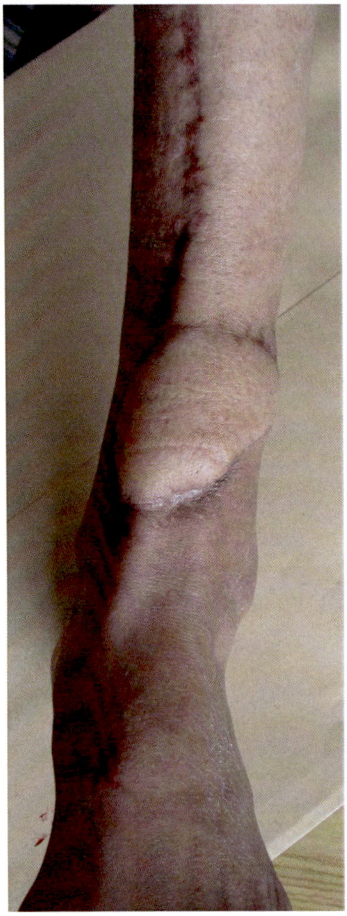

Fig. 25.19 Postoperative view

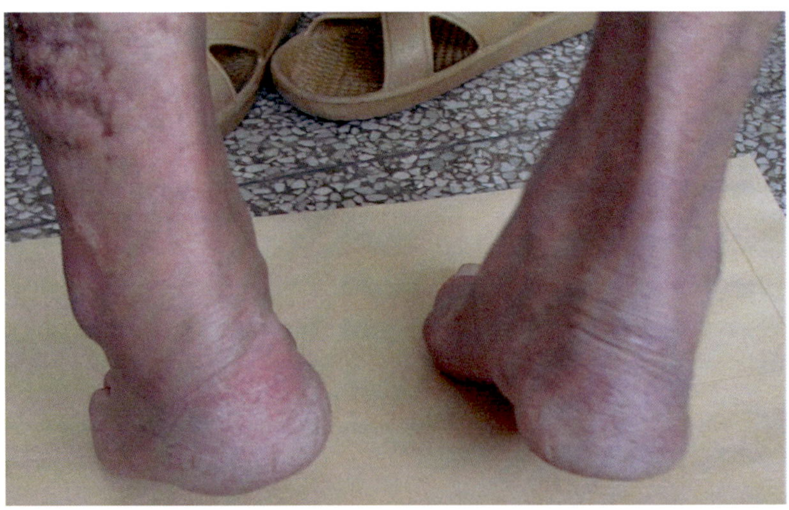

Fig. 25.20 Follow up

Pearls

It is a simple, rapid, one-stage procedure requiring no microsurgical technique.

It is easy to rotate the flap around the perforator.

Dog-ear deformity of the pedicle can be avoided.

It is a sufficiently large flap design and preserves the areolar tissue around the feeding perforator to prevent vascular kinking and stretching.

It moves the pivot point distally, thus reducing operative trauma and morbidity of the lower leg donor site.

No venous congestion was noted as the lesser saphenous vein was cut and ligated at both proximal and distal ends, which ruled out continuous venous ingress and engorgement through the distal base returned from the foot [3, 4].

Pitfalls

The skin island can never be outlined before the main perforating vessel is exposed. The skin incision should not be made over or lateral to the posterior intermuscular septum, because in this case the perforator will be missed. Preoperative mapping of the main perforator using an audible Doppler can facilitate planning the flap design.

The posterior intermuscular septum should be opened carefully to expose the perforator.

Especially in the common case of a myocutaneous perforator, these vessels must be carefully dissected on their course through the soleus and flexor hallucis muscles. Note that the cutaneous perforator regularly sends a branch to the peroneal muscles so that bleeding will occur when forming a small muscle cuff. Keep a distance of about 1 cm from the cutaneous branch to be able to cauterize the muscle bleeding without damaging the skin vessel.

The sural nerve and posterior saphenous vein may become exposed at the distolateral periphery of the skin flap and might be ligated, if necessary.

To facilitate elevation of the flap, hold the skin paddle between two fingers to protect the perforator from both sides. In case of a myocutaneous perforator, leave a small cuff of soleus muscle along the vessel, with its greatest thickness of about 1 cm around the perforator.

References

1. Aoki S, Tanuma K, Iwakiri I, et al. Clinical and vascular anatomical study of distally based sural flap. Ann Plast Surg. 2008;61(1):73–8.
2. Lecours C, Saint-Cyr M, Wong C, et al. Freestyle pedicle perforator flaps: clinical results and vascular anatomy. Plast Reconstr Surg. 2010;126(5):1589–603.
3. Chang SM, Gu YD, Li JF. Comparison of different managements of large superficial veins in distally based fasciocutaneous flaps with a veno-neuro-adipofascial pedicle: an experimental study using a rabbit model. Microsurgery. 2003;23(6):555–60.
4. Chang SM, Gu YD, Li JF. The role of the large superficial vein in survival of proximally based versus distally based sural veno-neuro-fasciocutaneous flaps in a rabbit model. Plast Reconstr Surg. 2005;115(1):213–8.

26 Medial Sural Artery Perforator Flap

The medial sural perforator flap was described in a very similar fashion in cadaver dissections by Taylor and Daniel [1] as a potential free flap donor site as early as 1975. Baek [2] was the first to report its clinical applications along with anatomical observations regarding medial and lateral femoral free flaps. The true medial sural perforator free flap was first introduced by Cavadas et al. [3].

26.1 Vascular Anatomy

The medial sural artery arises from the popliteal artery and, after running 2–5 cm, enters the deep surface of the medial gastrocnemius muscle. Within the muscle, the medial sural artery may be either a dominant vascular pedicle or may divide into two branches that run longitudinally between the muscle fiber bundles and give off musculocutaneous perforators to the overlying skin [4, 5].

The medial sural artery runs along an imaginary line connecting the midpoint of the popliteal crease and the midpoint of the medial malleolus.

At least one large musculocutaneous perforator exits through the medial head of the gastrocnemius muscle to allow the creation of a true perforator flap using the overlying calf skin territory. The majority of these perforators are clustered in the distal half of the muscle and emanate near the raphe separating the two heads of the gastrocnemius [6, 7].

C. Hou et al., *Surgical Atlas of Perforator Flaps: A Microsurgical Dissection Technique*,
DOI 10.1007/978-94-017-9834-1_26, © Springer Science+Business Media Dordrecht 2015

26.2 Illustrative Case

A 37-year-old woman suffered a crushing injury to the medial side of her right lower leg, with overlying soft tissue loss measured 6.5 × 5.0 cm (Fig. 26.2).

Flap Design

The design of the desired flap is centered around the most distal perforator found to ensure the longest possible pedicle (Fig. 26.3). The main perforators of the medial sural artery are located on a line drawn from the midpoint of the popliteal crease to the midpoint of the medial malleolus. Using an audible Doppler probe to locate a distal perforator over the medial calf, a template of the defect was then centered about this point to create a 6.5 × 4.2 cm flap (Fig. 26.4).

Flap Elevation

The lateral and/or distal border of the flap is first raised to confirm the location and size of the perforators (Fig. 26.5). Next, an intramuscular dissection of the identified perforator through the medial gastrocnemius muscle proceeds back to the medial sural vessels to obtain the desired pedicle length. The remaining boundaries of the flap are incised through the deep fascia (Fig. 26.6).

The flap was rotated 180° to cover the defect. The donor site was closed directly (Fig. 26.7).

Follow-Up

The flap survived well and allowed unrestricted ambulation, and a linear scar of the donor area was obtained 3 months postoperatively (Fig. 26.8).

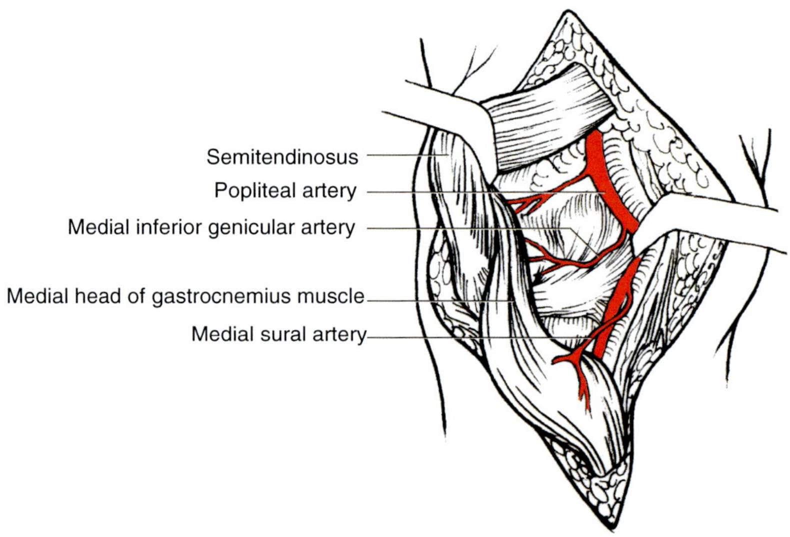

Fig. 26.1 Vascular anatomy of the medial sural artery

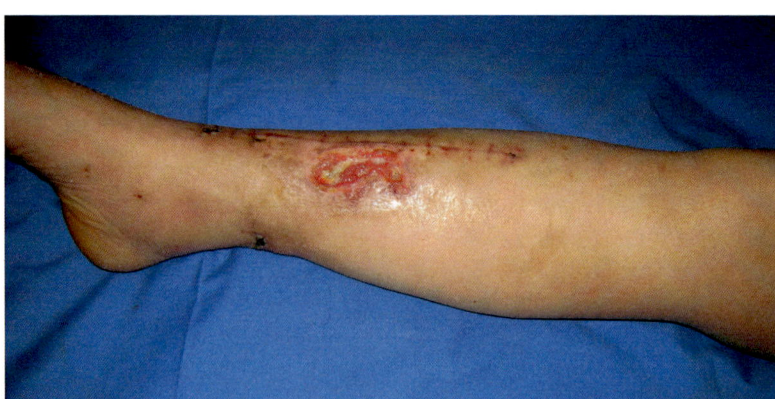

Fig. 26.2 Preoperative view

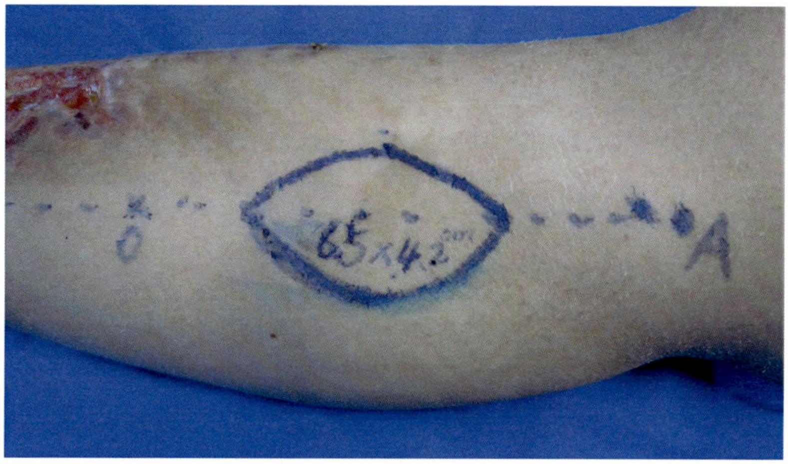

Fig. 26.3 Flap design

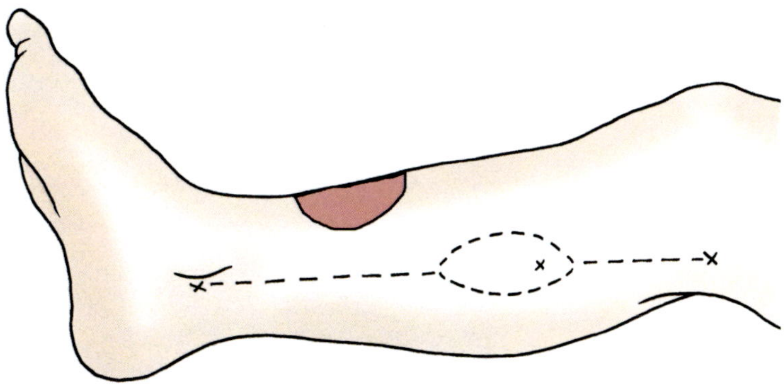

Fig. 26.4 Schematic drawing of flap design

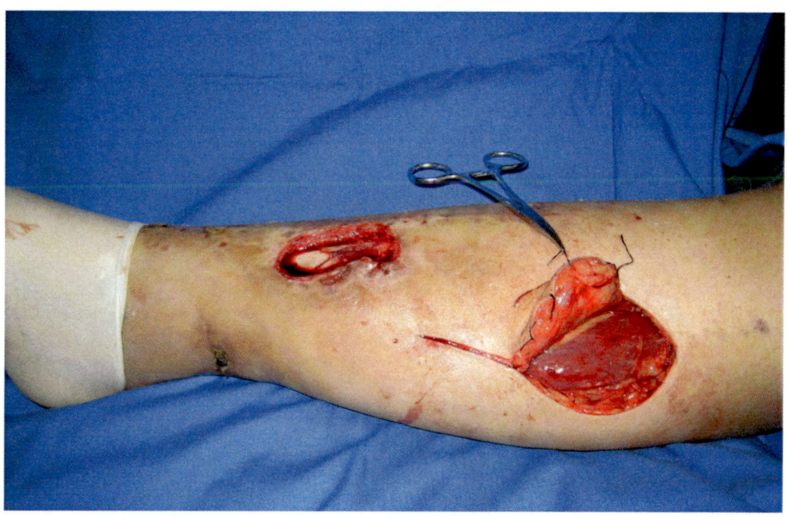

Fig. 26.5 Perforator vessel visualization

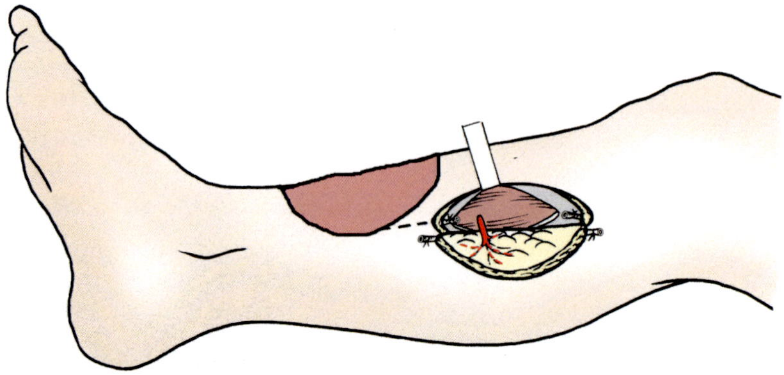

Fig. 26.6 Schematic drawing of the flap elevation

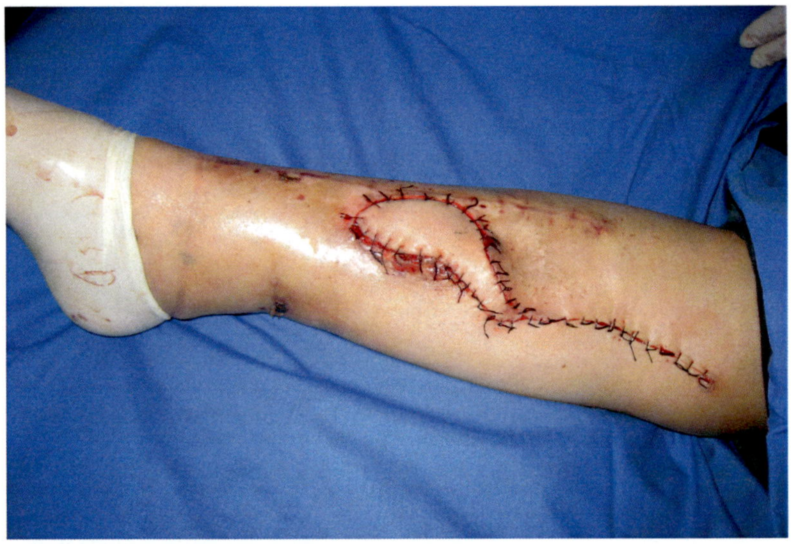

Fig. 26.7 Flap transfer and insetting

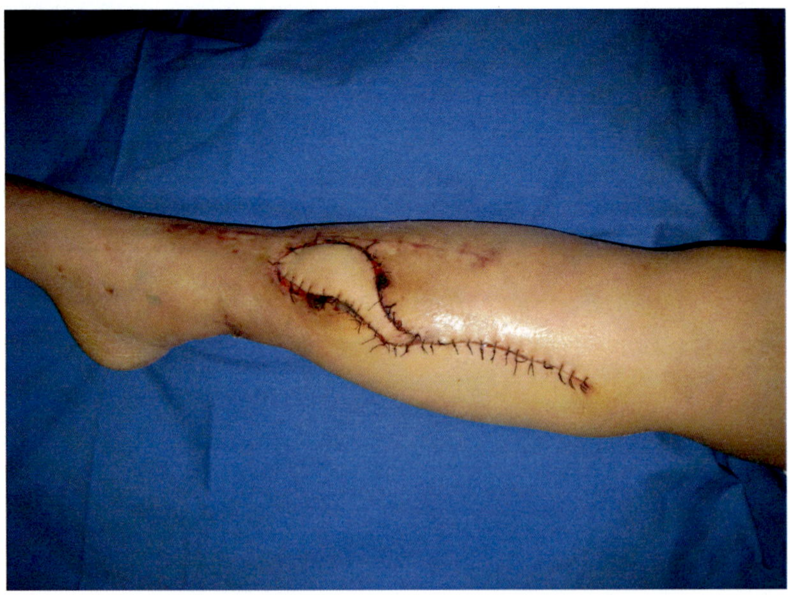

Fig. 26.8 Follow-up

Pearls

The medial sural perforator flap, also called medial gastrocnemius flap, is a potentially large, thin cutaneous flap [8–11].

Its medial sural vascular pedicle has a long leash of large caliber [12–14].

Pitfalls

Use of a tourniquet without exsanguinations of the leg facilitates the dissection [15].

During the flap dissection, if these are reasonable, the remaining boundaries of the flap are incised through the deep fascia, preserving a proximal superficial vein for another source of outflow if the deep veins later prove to be inadequate [16].

Occasionally, a medial sural perforator flap will not be anatomically feasible, because the gastrocnemius musculocutaneous perforators could instead have their origin from the superficial median sural artery or be too diminutive [17–19].

References

1. Taylor GI, Daniel RK. The anatomy of several free flap donor sites. Plast Reconstr Surg. 1975;56(3):243–53.
2. Baek SM. Two new cutaneous free flaps: the medial and lateral thigh flaps. Plast Reconstr Surg. 1983;71(3):354–65.
3. Cavadas PC, Sanz-Gimenez-Rico JR, Gutierrez-de la Camara A, Navarro-Monzonis A, Soler-Nomdedeu S, Martinez-Soriano F. The medial sural artery perforator free flap. Plast Reconstr Surg. 2001;108(6):1609–15; discussion 1616–1607.
4. Potparic Z, Colen LB, Sucur D, Carwell GR, Carraway JH. The gastrocnemius muscle as a free-flap donor site. Plast Reconstr Surg. 1995;95(7):1245–52.
5. Hallock GG. Anatomic basis of the gastrocnemius perforator-based flap. Ann Plast Surg. 2001;47(5):517–22.
6. Al-Qattan MM. A modified technique for harvesting the reverse sural artery flap from the upper part of the leg: inclusion of a gastrocnemius muscle "cuff" around the sural pedicle. Ann Plast Surg. 2001;47(3):269–74, discussion 274–268.
7. Wen G, Chai Y, Wang C, Wu X, Wang L, Cheng L. [Study on animal model of perforator sural neurocutaneous flap]. Zhongguo xiu fu chong jian wai ke za zhi = Zhongguo xiufu chongjian waike zazhi = Chin J Reparative Reconstr Surg. 2010;24(4):458–61.
8. He Y, Jin SF, Zhang ZY, Feng SQ, Zhang CP, Zhang YX. A prospective study of medial sural artery perforator flap with computed tomographic angiography-aided design in tongue reconstruction. J Oral Maxillofac Surg Off J Am Assoc Oral Maxillofac Surg. 2014;72(11):2351–65.
9. Zhu YL, Wang Y, He XQ, Zhu M, Li FB, Xu YQ. Foot and ankle reconstruction: an experience on the use of 14 different flaps in 226 cases. Microsurgery. 2013;24(2):127–31.
10. Mao C, Zhang L, Cui QJ, Peng X, Wang Y, Yu GY. [A preliminary study on free medial sural artery perforator flap for head and neck reconstruction following tumor ablation]. Zhonghua kou qiang yi xue za zhi = Zhonghua kouqiang yixue zazhi = Chin J Stomatol. 2011;46(12):742–6.
11. Xie XT, Chai YM. Medial sural artery perforator flap. Ann Plast Surg. 2012;68(1):105–10.
12. Hallock GG. Medial sural artery perforator free flap: legitimate use as a solution for the ipsilateral distal lower extremity defect. J Reconstr Microsurg. 2014;30(3):187–92.
13. Xie RG, Gu JH, Gong YP, Tang JB. Medial sural artery perforator flap for repair of the hand. J Hand Surg Eur Vol. 2007;32(5):512–7.
14. Xia HC, An Y, Hou ZJ, Xia SY, Fu ZP, Zhang GQ. [Clinical application of sural neurocutaneous island flaps]. Zhonghua zheng xing wai ke za zhi = Zhonghua zhengxing waike zazhi = Chin J Plast Surg. 2006;22(4):256–8.
15. Cui Y, Cai J, Liu L, et al. [Repair of wounds with Achilles tendon exposure]. Zhongguo xiu fu chong jian wai ke za zhi = Zhongguo xiufu chongjian waike zazhi = Chin J Reparative Reconstr Surg. 2011;25(5):565–8.
16. Lin CH, Lin YT, Hsu CC, Ng TW, Wei FC. The medial sural artery perforator flap: a versatile donor site for hand reconstruction. J Trauma. 2011;70(3):736–43.
17. Shaw AD, Ghosh SJ, Quaba AA. The island posterior calf fasciocutaneous flap: an alternative to the gastrocnemius muscle for cover of knee and tibial defects. Plast Reconstr Surg. 1998;101(6):1529–36.
18. Wang X, Mei J, Pan J, Chen H, Zhang W, Tang M. Reconstruction of distal limb defects with the free medial sural artery perforator flap. Plast Reconstr Surg. 2013;131(1):95–105.
19. Wei ZR, Shao X, Xie Y, et al. [Repair of wounds in popliteal fossa scar with perforator flaps of gastrocnemius medial head]. Zhonghua shao shang za zhi = Zhonghua shaoshang zazhi = Chin J Burns. 2010;26(4):260–2.

Peroneal Artery Anterolateral Supramalleolar Flap

27

The distally based lateral supramalleolar flap, nourished by the supramalleolar anterior perforating branch of the peroneal artery, was firstly reported by Masquelet in 1988 [1]. The flap was then modified by other researchers to reach more distal region such as the forefoot defect.

27.1 Vascular Anatomy

The anterolateral supramalleolar flap is based on the anterior perforating branch of the peroneal artery, which pierces the intermuscular septum and appears on the front of the leg approximately 5 cm above the lateral malleolus. Here it divides into 2 branches, one is a deep branch which runs distally in the loose areolar fatty tissue under the deep fascia (retinaculum), running over the tarsal bones and anastomosing with other vessels, such as the branches of the anterior tibial artery, dorsalis pedis artery, and the terminal part of the peroneal artery which is called lateral calcaneal artery. The other branch is a superficial cutaneous branch, which emerges between the extensor digitorum longus and the peroneus brevis muscles and expended in proximal direction.

The flap pedicle can be designed in 2 versions. One is based on the perforating point with a local transposition for malleolar defect. The second is based on the distal anastomosis; the flap is perfused from the deep branch to the main trunk and then to the superficial cutaneous branch [2]. The second version is for more distal defect such as the forefoot (Fig. 27.1).

C. Hou et al., *Surgical Atlas of Perforator Flaps: A Microsurgical Dissection Technique*,
DOI 10.1007/978-94-017-9834-1_27, © Springer Science+Business Media Dordrecht 2015

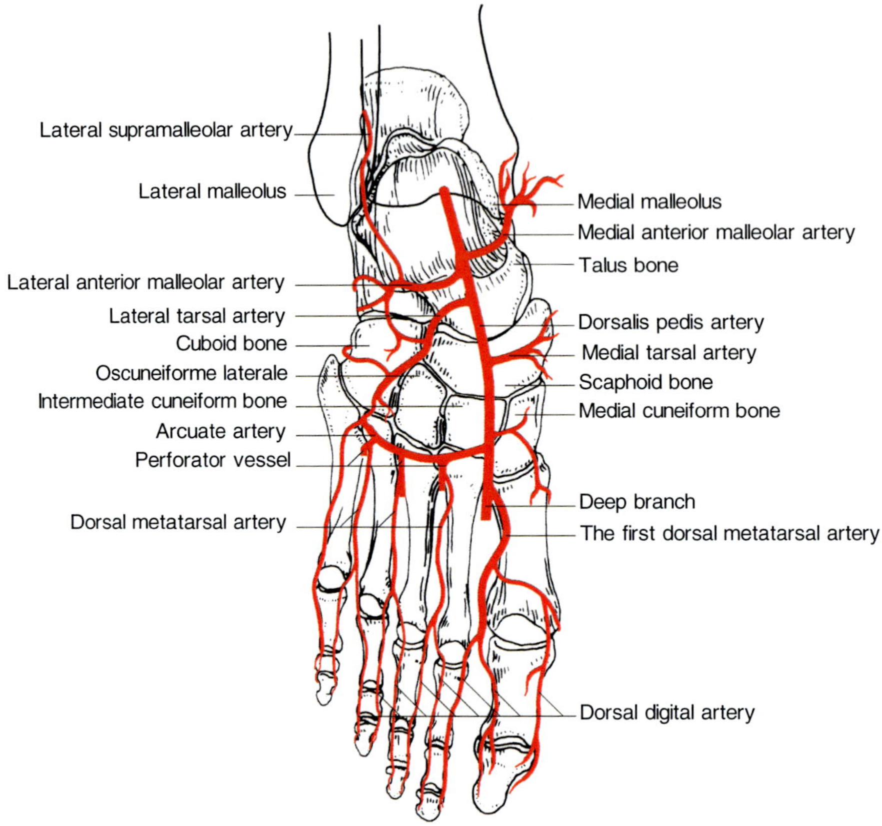

Fig. 27.1 Vascular anatomy of anterolateral supramalleolar flap

27.2 Illustrative Case

A 35-year-old man suffered a traffic accident which caused an open fracture of his right foot over the fifth metatarsal bone and a soft-tissue defect (Fig. 27.2). After primary debridement, the wound became clean and a distally based supramalleolar flap was designed to cover the defect, which is nourished by the axial anastomosis between the descending deep branch and the anterior tibial artery located at the tarsal sinus (Fig. 27.3).

A distal movement of the pivot point (e.g., 4 cm) reduces the length of the designed flap (in 8 cm), thus minimizing the morbidity of the lower leg donor site (Fig. 27.4).

The anterior perforating vessel bundle of the peroneal artery in the anterolateral septum, which was located 5 cm above the lateral malleolus (Fig. 27.5).

An axial anastomosis between the deep descending branch and the anterior tibial artery was located 1 cm above the malleolar tip. The flap got blood perfusion from the anterior tibial artery, through the deep descending branch to the main trunk and then to the superficial branch to the flap (Fig. 27.6).

The flap (skin paddle 12×6 cm) was rotated 180° to reach the recipient site through a 6 cm pedicle. Partial donor site was skin grafted. The flap showed good vascularization (Fig. 27.7).

The flap and skin graft showed full survival (Fig. 27.8).

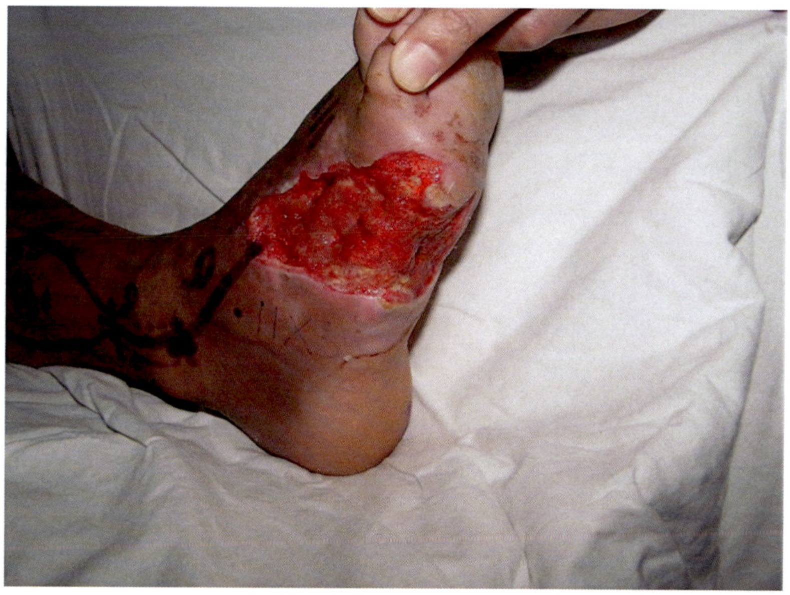

Fig. 27.2 The lateral forefoot wound measured 11×5 cm

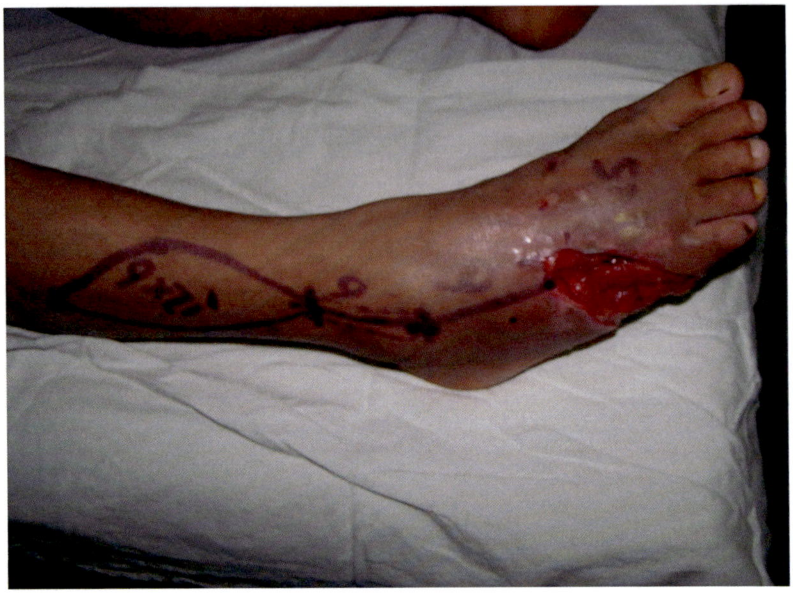

Fig. 27.3 The supramalleolar flap measured 12×6 cm in size. The estimated pedicle length is 6 cm

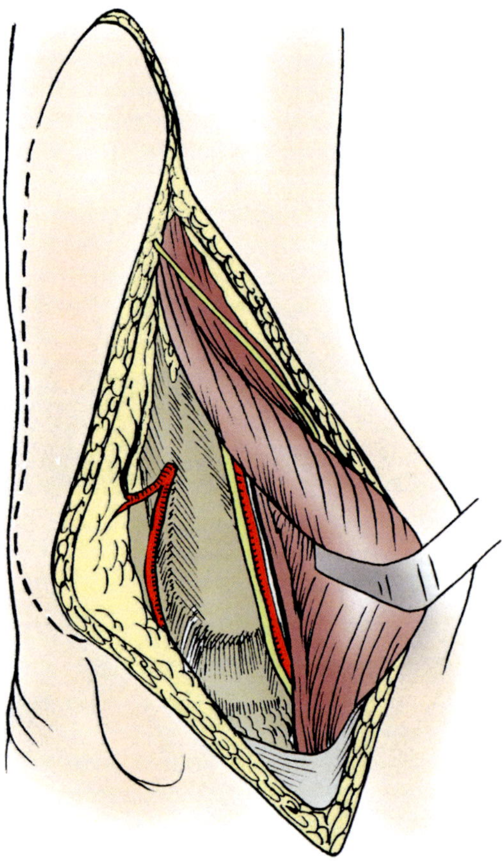

Fig. 27.4 Schematic drawing to show the flap design

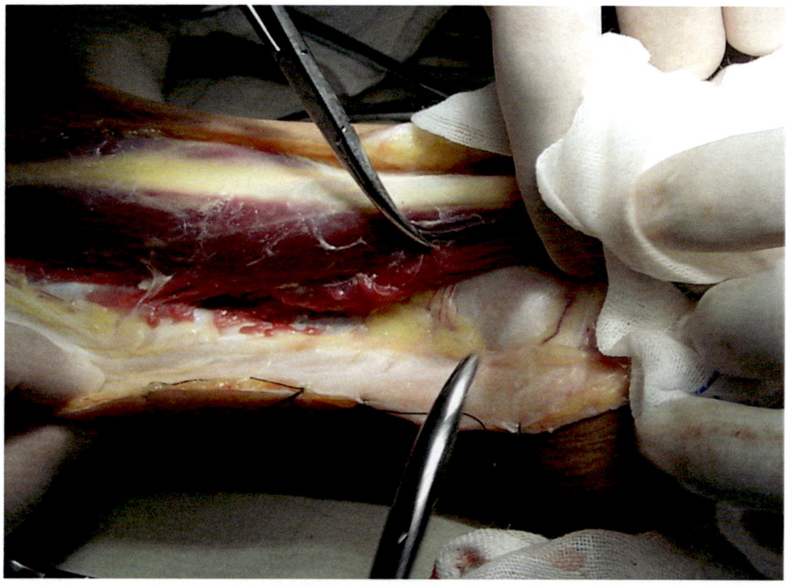

Fig. 27.5 Perforator vessel visualization

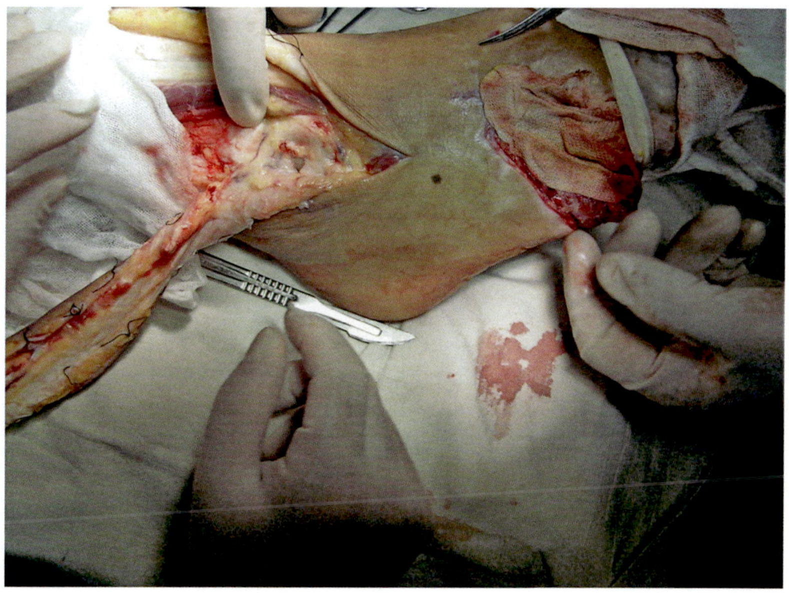

Fig. 27.6 Flap transfer

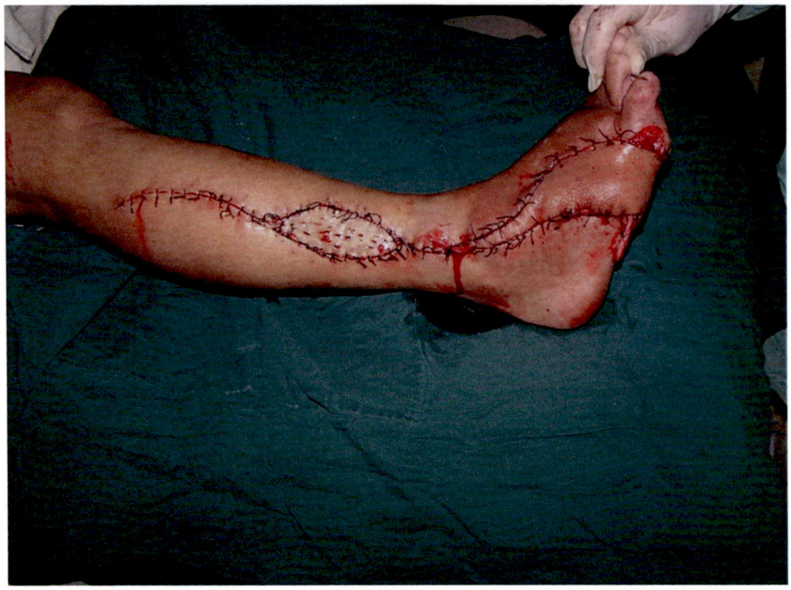

Fig. 27.7 Flap insetting

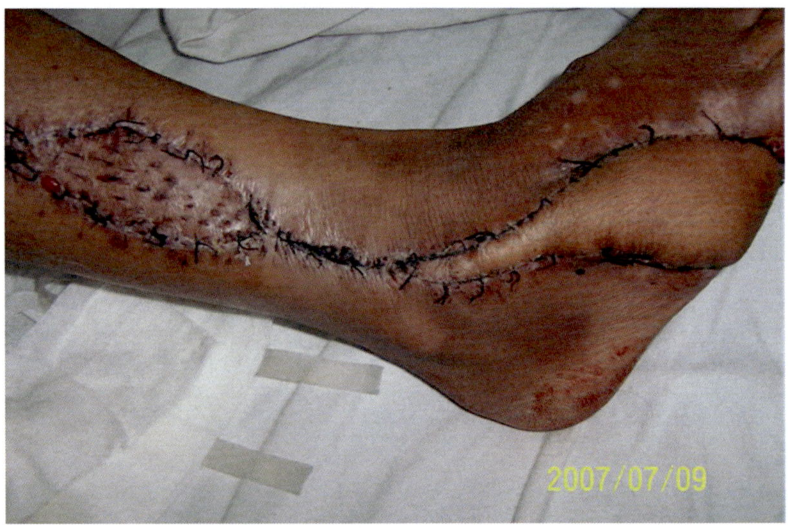

Fig. 27.8 Follow-up

Pearls

The distally based lateral supramalleolar flap has the advantages of both an axial perforator of the pedicle and the longitudinal chain-linked vascular plexuses of the neurofasciocutaneous flap, which allows safe elevation of a long flap.

The advantages of the flap include the following:

1. It is a simple, rapid, one-stage procedure requiring no microsurgical technique.
2. It is easy to rotate the flap around the perforator.
3. Dog-ear deformity of the pedicle can be avoided.
4. It is a sufficient flap design for small- to medium-sized defect (<10 cm).

References

1. Masquelet AC, Beveridge J, Romana C, et al. The lateral supramalleolar flap. Plast Reconstr Surg. 1988;81:74–81.
2. Valenti P, Masquelet AC, Romana C, et al. Technical refinement of the lateral supramalleolar flap. Br J Plast Surg. 1991;44:459–62.

Anterior Supramalleolar Perforator Flap

28

The anterior supramalleolar perforator flap is pedicled on the superior malleolar cutaneous branch of the anterior tibial artery. It is a fasciocutaneous flap located in the middle-distal third of the lower leg.

A variant of adipofacial flaps based on perforators of the distal anterior tibial artery have been used to cover complex ankle defects [1, 2].

28.1 Vascular Anatomy

Anatomic dissections of cadaveric legs demonstrated a constant dominant perforator located 3.5 cm above the line between the medial malleolus and lateral malleolus. There was no significant branching pattern variability noted, except at the subdermal level (Fig. 28.1).

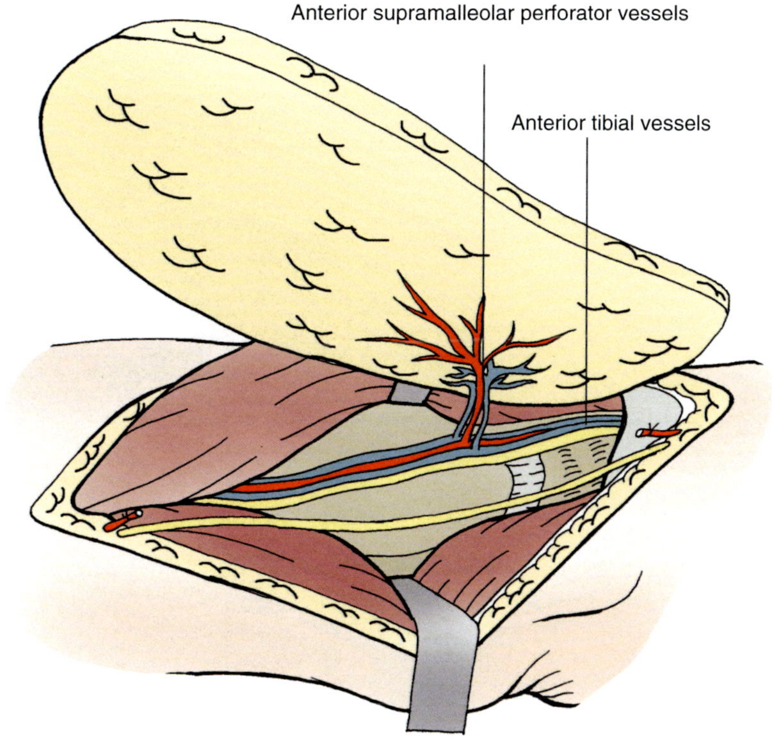

Fig. 28.1 Vascular anatomy of the anterior supramalleolar perforator flap

C. Hou et al., *Surgical Atlas of Perforator Flaps: A Microsurgical Dissection Technique*,
DOI 10.1007/978-94-017-9834-1_28, © Springer Science+Business Media Dordrecht 2015

28.2 Illustrative Case

A 45-year-old male suffered a traffic accident over his right dorsal foot, resulting in skin and soft tissue defect, with exposure of the dorsal bones and tendons (Fig. 28.2).

Flap Design

The wound was covered with a distally pedicled flap based on anterior tibial artery perforators.

A handheld ultrasound Doppler scanner was used preoperatively to detect perforator arteries around the donor-site area, and a free-style perforator flap was used (Fig. 28.3).

The flap was planned according to the position and size of the defect, taking into account the need to avoid excessive tension on the border of the propeller flap during suturing (Fig. 28.4).

Flap Elevation

A dissection was initiated at the subfascial level from the posterior side of the designed flap outline along the anterolateral direction and continued to the perforator point. Perforator artery selection before flap harvesting was based on vessel size and distance to the area of the defect.

The flap was redesigned centering movement of propeller blades around the point at which the perforator artery emerged from fascia. Then, the dissection was performed in the same way on the anterior side. When reaching the septocutaneous perforator, the dissection proceeded deeply along the anterior intermuscular septum between the extensor digitorum longus and tibialis anterior or peroneus longus (Fig. 28.5).

After confirming the perforator as a branch of the ATA, the perforator vessel was dissected back to the ATA, leaving a small piece of fascia encircling the perforator. The ATA perforator was traced until a sufficient length was obtained.

Flap Transfer

The flap was then rotated 180° to reach the recipient site (Fig. 28.6).

Postoperative view with the propeller flap rotated 180° around the perforator vessel.

After propeller rotation, the minor skin paddle helped the closure of the donor site.

Skin grafts were required to cover the secondary defect, as direct closure was not possible (Fig. 28.7)

Follow-Up

Aesthetic result in follow-up 4 months (Fig. 28.8)

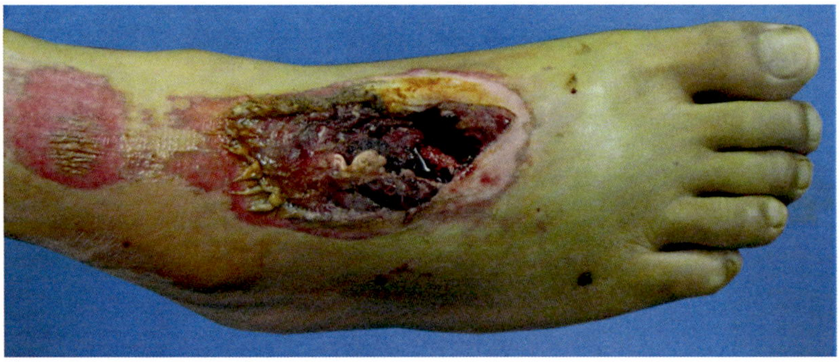

Fig. 28.2 Preoperative view

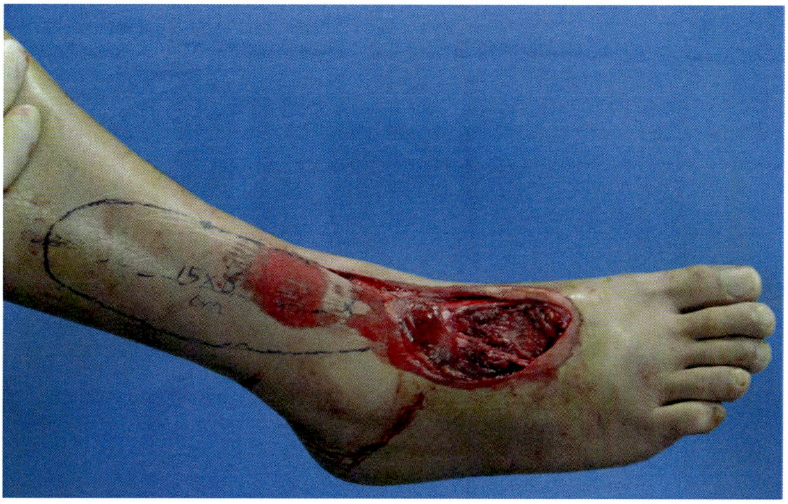

Fig. 28.3 Flap design

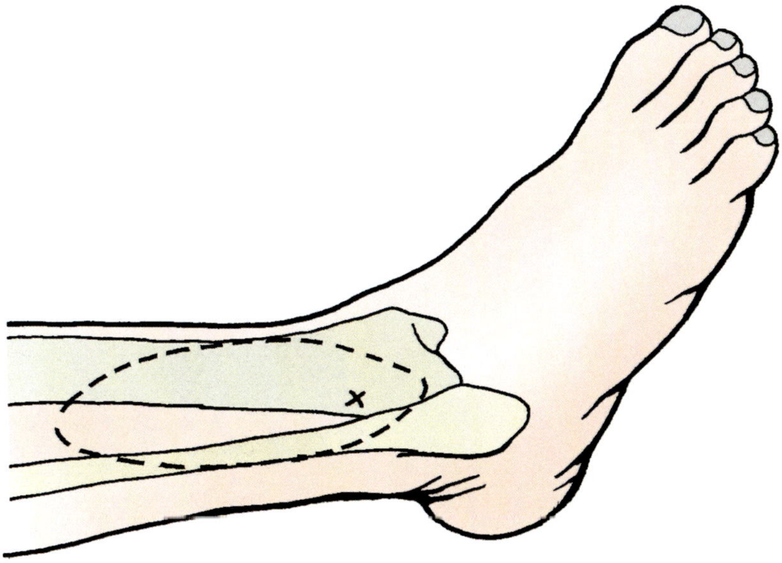

Fig. 28.4 Schematic drawing of flap design

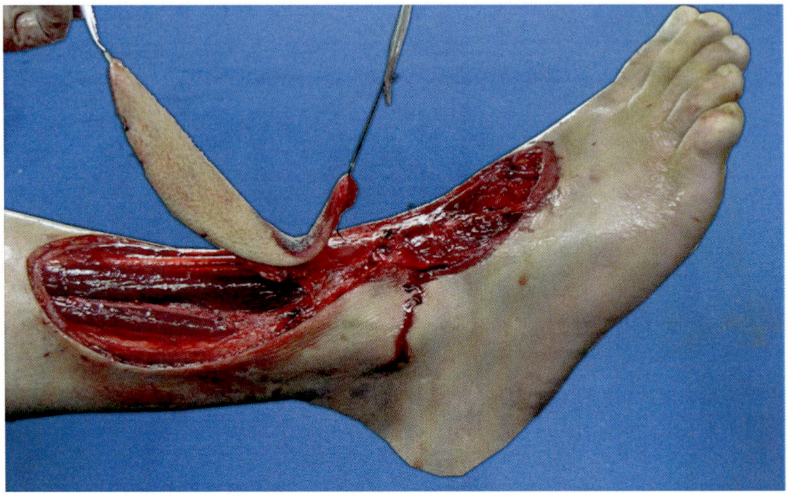

Fig. 28.5 Flap elevation

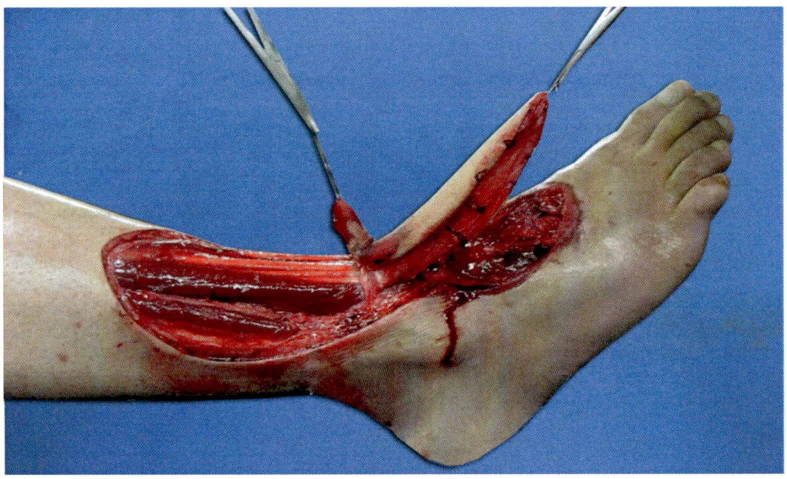

Fig. 28.6 Flap rotation

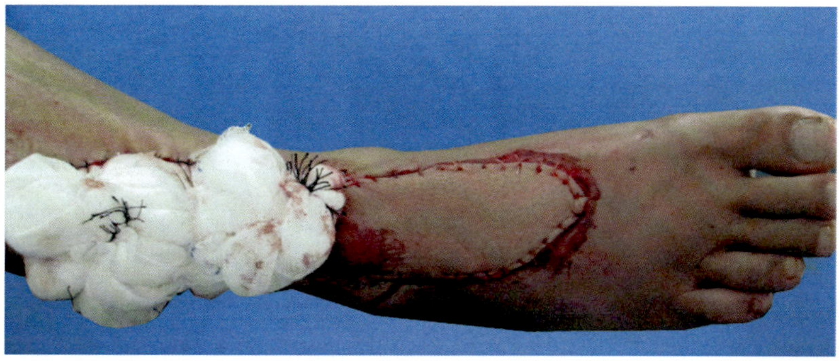

Fig. 28.7 Postoperative view

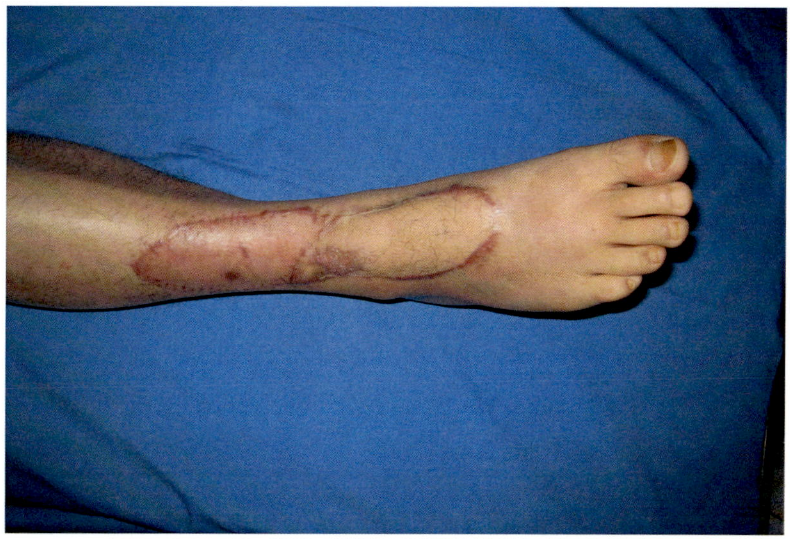

Fig. 28.8 Follow-up

Pearls

The main advantages of the ATAP flap are its thin and pliable tissue characteristics.

For small- and medium-sized defects, the ATAP flap is a reliable alternative to the free flap.

If possible, direct closure of the donor site was performed without tension on the edge of the flap.

When closure was performed using a skin graft, immobilization for 10 days was prescribed.

Retrograde intramuscular dissection of the principal perforator maximizes pedicle length. This distributes the 180° rotation over a greater pedicle length and minimizes tension and twist on the pedicle.

Inclusion of a fascia into the flap depended on the donor site and the characteristics of the lesion.

Pitfalls

Manipulation was performed carefully to avoid injury to the deep peroneal nerve.

During the dissection procedure, particular attention was paid to preserve the vascular pedicle. Vascular-pedicle traction during flap harvesting and positioning was carefully avoided.

Bandaging was soft, to avoid compression over the flap, and the limb was held in an elevated position.

References

1. Kilinc H, Bilen BT, Arslan A. A novel flap to repair medial and lateral malleolar defects: anterior tibial artery perforator-based adipofascial flap. Ann Plast Surg. 2006;57(4):396–401.
2. Recalde Rocha JF, Gilbert A, Masquelet A, Yousif NJ, Sanger JR, Matloub HS. The anterior tibial artery flap: anatomic study and clinical application. Plast Reconstr Surg. 1987;79(3):396–406.

29 Medial Supramalleolar Perforator Flap

The medial supramalleolar perforator flap has proved an excellent option for the coverage of soft tissue defects in the lower third of the leg, ankle, and foot [1–6].

29.1 Vascular Anatomy

In the medial aspect of the leg, some perforators from the posterior tibial artery are located in the medial aspect of the lower leg and the medial plantar region. Perforators from the posterior tibial artery emerge at periodic intervals between the soleus and flexor digitorum longus muscles. The medial supramalleolar perforator, located 5 cm above the medial malleolus, supplies the medial supramalleolar perforator flap (Fig. 29.1).

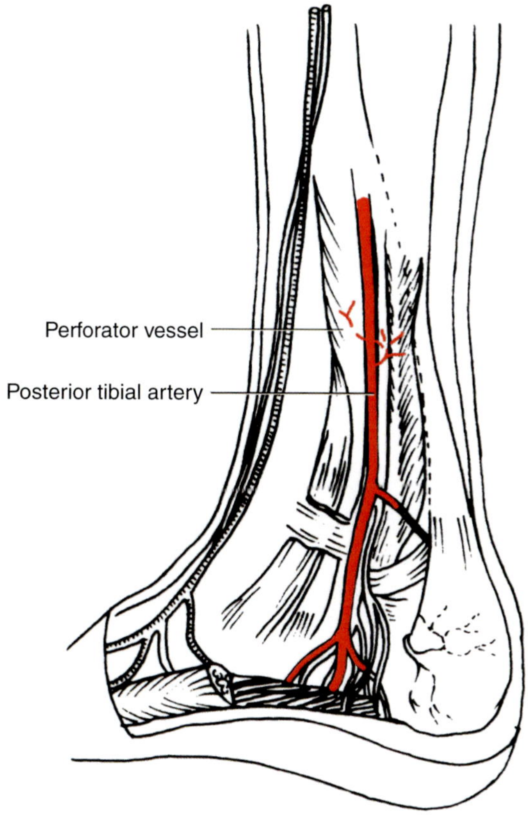

Fig. 29.1 Vascular anatomy of the medial supramalleolar perforator flap

C. Hou et al., *Surgical Atlas of Perforator Flaps: A Microsurgical Dissection Technique*,
DOI 10.1007/978-94-017-9834-1_29, © Springer Science+Business Media Dordrecht 2015

29.2 Illustrative Case

A 56-year-old man sustained a traffic accident injury on his left foot. The resulting wound measured 13×4 cm (Fig. 29.2).

Flap Design

According to the location of the defect, perforators of the posterior tibial vessels were preoperatively selected and marked with a handheld Doppler device. All perforators proximal to the defect were marked, with special attention to the dominant vessel (Fig. 29.3). The flap was designed based on the location of the pivot point of the major perforator. A line was drawn from the malleolus to the medial tibial condyle. The flap was then outlined and centered on this line according to the size of the tissue defect (Fig. 29.4).

An incision was made along the posterior border of the flap. The terminal posterior tibial perforating vessel was located in the fascial plexus of the flap by careful dissection. During the dissection procedure, particular attention was paid to preserve the vascular pedicle (Fig. 29.5).

The great saphenous vein and saphenous nerve traveled through the proposed flap; they were dissected out and left intact (Fig. 29.6). Dissection of both the vein and nerve was carried out under loupe magnification; the accompanying vessels were divided meticulously from the great saphenous vein and saphenous nerve and included in the flap. The flap was completely elevated and was attached to the donor site only with the perforating vessels (Fig. 29.7).

With only the terminal posterior tibial perforating branch as the pedicle, the flap was raised in an island form above the deep fascia. The flap was then rotated 150° to reach the recipient site (Fig. 29.8).

The patient was satisfied with the functional and esthetic results (Fig. 29.9).

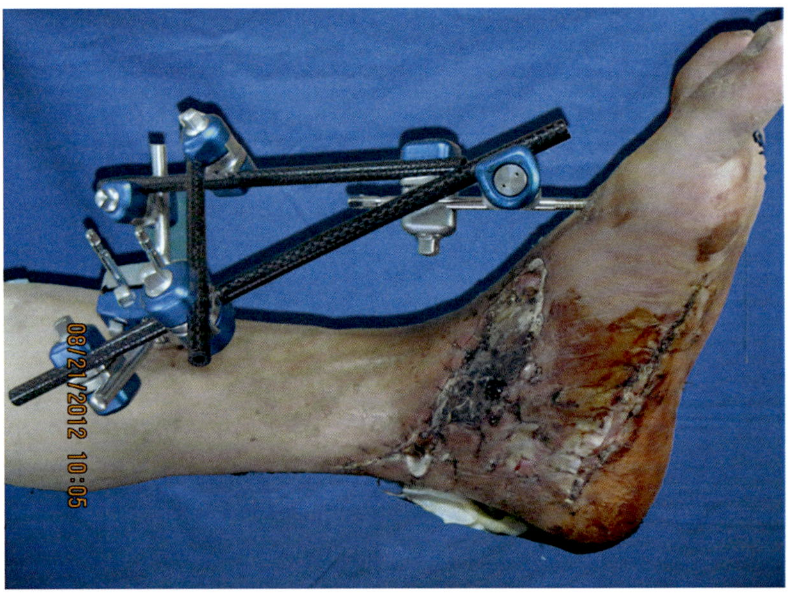

Fig. 29.2 Preoperative view

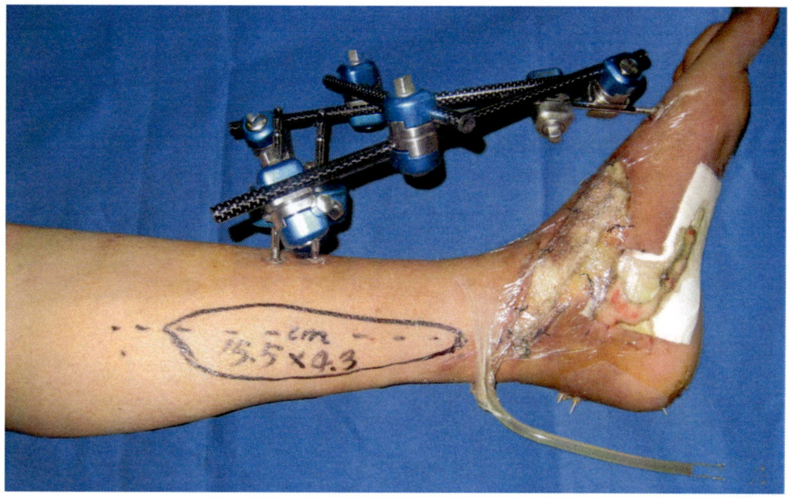

Fig. 29.3 Flap design

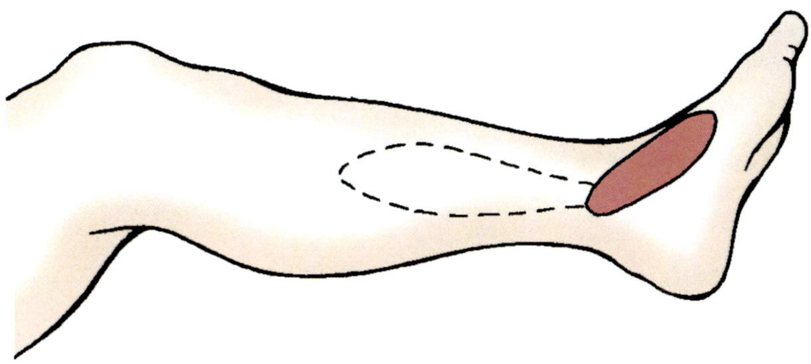

Fig. 29.4 Schematic drawing of flap design

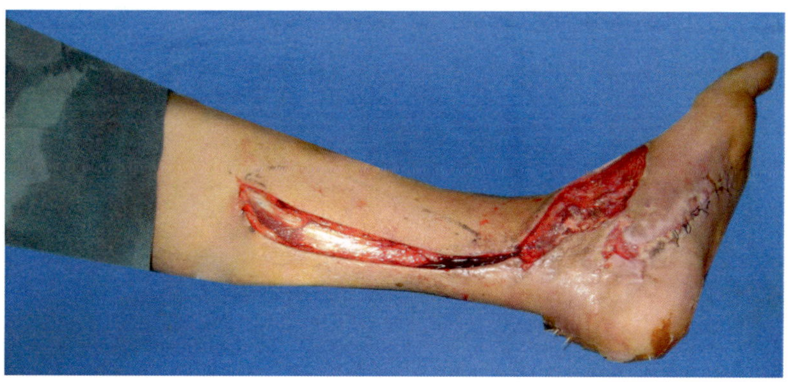

Fig. 29.5 Perforator vessel visualization

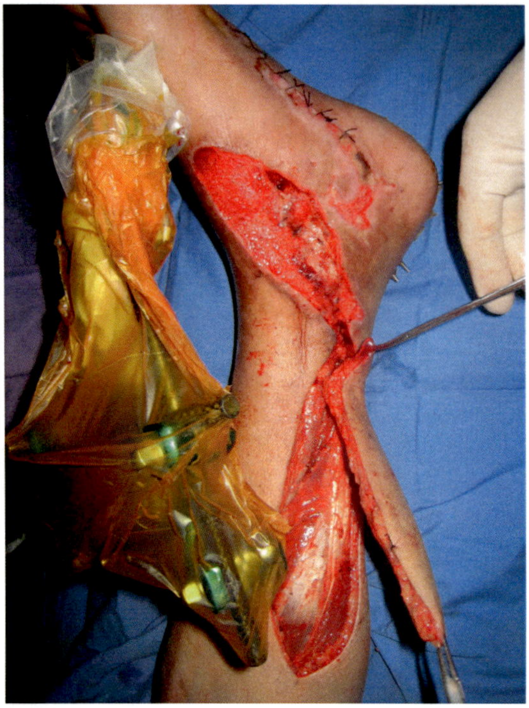

Fig. 29.6 Flap elevation

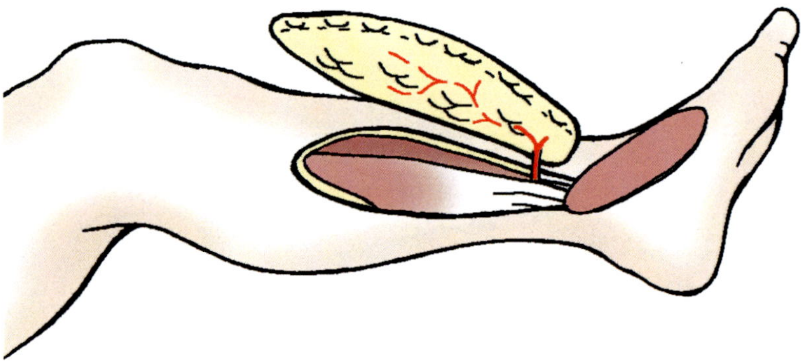

Fig. 29.7 Schematic drawing of the flap elevation

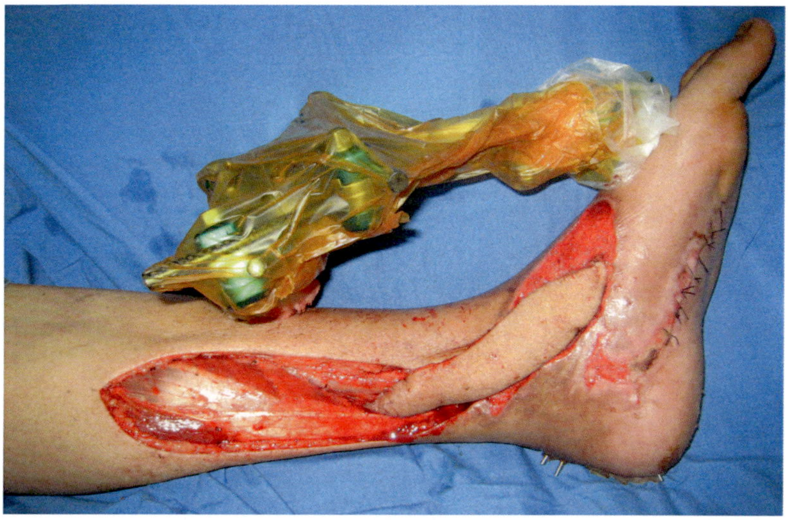

Fig. 29.8 Flap transfer and insetting

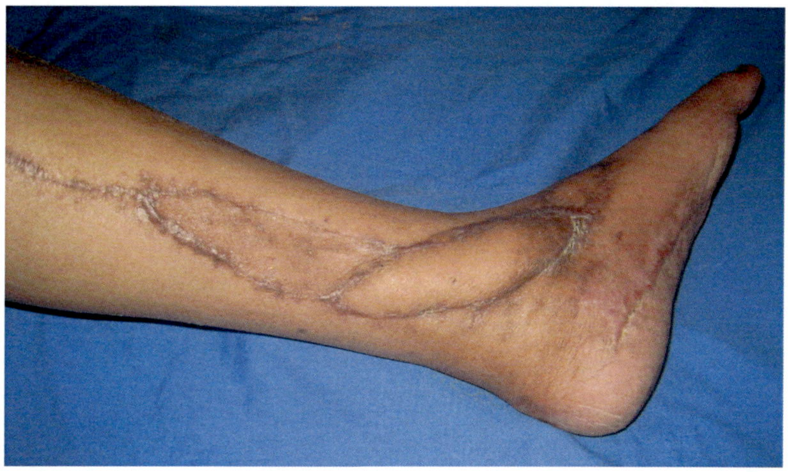

Fig. 29.9 Postoperative view

Pearls

Flap harvest is relatively quick, and the recipient site has similar texture, thickness, pliability, and pigmentation to that which has been lost.

V-Y or propeller flap designs may enable primary closure. These flaps are particularly suitable for complicated defects of the lower third of the leg, foot, heel, and ankle.

Pitfalls

Preoperative examination with a Doppler probe can help prevent damage to the terminal perforating branch of the posterior tibial artery.

Perforator artery selection before flap harvesting was based on vessel size and distance to the area of the defect. Once an artery with an adequate caliber and venae comitantes have been verified clinically, the flap design may have to be reevaluated. If the location of the main perforator does not correlate with the anticipated pivot point, the flap design must be adapted accordingly.

References

1. Cavadas PC, Landin L. Reconstruction of chronic Achilles tendon defects with posterior tibial perforator flap and soleus tendon graft: clinical series. Plast Reconstr Surg. 2006;117(1):266–71.
2. Foo TL, Chew WY, Tan BK. Improving the reliability of the distally based posterior tibial artery adipofascial flap with the great saphenous venoneural network. Ann Plast Surg. 2011;67(3):288–93.
3. Ozdemir R, Kocer U, Sahin B, Oruc M, Kilinc H, Tekdemir I. Examination of the skin perforators of the posterior tibial artery on the leg and the ankle region and their clinical use. Plast Reconstr Surg. 2006;117(5):1619–30.
4. Parrett BM, Winograd JM, Lin SJ, Borud LJ, Taghinia A, Lee BT. The posterior tibial artery perforator flap: an alternative to free-flap closure in the comorbid patient. J Reconstr Microsurg. 2009;25(2):105–9.
5. Robotti E, Carminati M, Bonfirraro PP, et al. "On demand" posterior tibial artery perforator flaps: a versatile surgical procedure for reconstruction of soft tissue defects of the leg after tumor excision. Ann Plast Surg. 2010;64(2):202–9.
6. Schaverien M, Saint-Cyr M. Perforators of the lower leg: analysis of perforator locations and clinical application for pedicled perforator flaps. Plast Reconstr Surg. 2008;122(1):161–70.

30 Dorsal Metatarsal Artery Perforator Flap

Earley and Milner [1] described distally based first web flaps that included branches of the first dorsal and plantar metatarsal arteries and which they used to cover distal dorsal foot defects.

The reverse first dorsal metatarsal artery (FDMA) flap has a longer vascular pedicle and can be used for distal foot wounds [2].

30.1 Vascular Anatomy

The dorsalis pedis artery, which is an extension of the anterior tibial artery, supplies the flap. The anterior tibial artery lies lateral to the tibialis anterior tendon and medial to the extensor hallucis longus tendon at the entrance of the extensor retinaculum or the ankle. It courses under the retinaculum and emerges medial to the extensor hallucis longus tendon as the dorsalis pedis artery. The dorsalis pedis artery branches to form the arcuate artery and lateral and medial tarsal arteries, which supply structures beneath the extensor tendons and are not harvested as part of the flap [3–5].

The artery branches into the first dorsal metatarsal artery and deep perforating branch at the first intermetatarsal space. The critical point, where the first dorsal metatarsal artery (or the first plantar metatarsal artery in cases when the former branched from the latter) was located 10 mm distal to the tarsal-first metatarsal joint and 5.5 mm plantar from the dorsal surface of the second metatarsal bone (Fig. 30.1).

C. Hou et al., *Surgical Atlas of Perforator Flaps: A Microsurgical Dissection Technique*,
DOI 10.1007/978-94-017-9834-1_30,

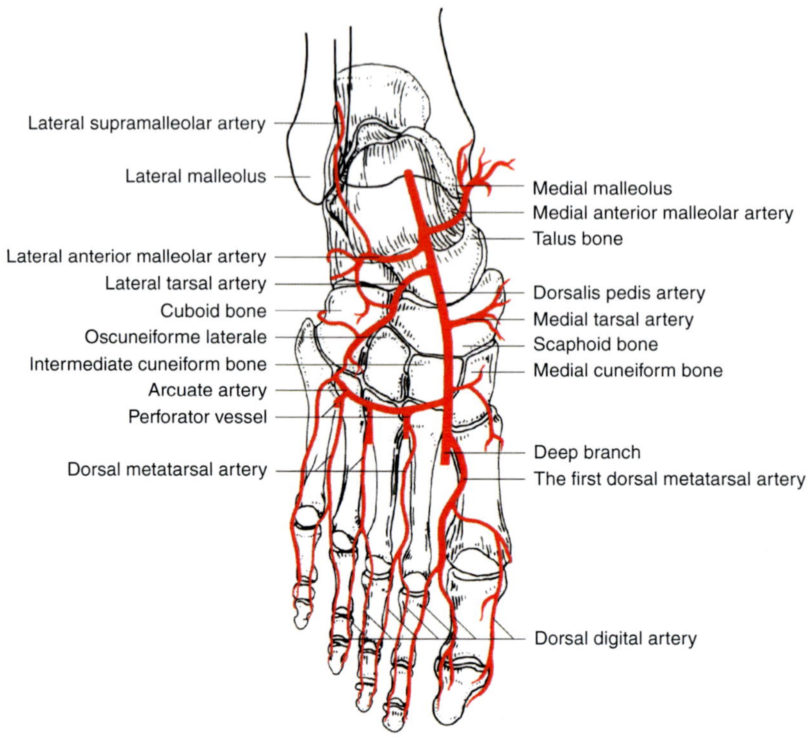

Fig. 30.1 Vascular anatomy of the dorsalis pedis artery

30.2 Illustrative Case

A 32-year-old man presented with a press injury over his distal portion of the foot and big toe, with skin and soft tissue necrosis. A thorough debridement was carried out, leaving a defect of 4.5 cm × 2.0 cm over the big toe (Fig. 30.2).

Flap Design

A preoperative Doppler examination evaluates the blood flow of dorsalis pedis artery, the plantar artery, and the FDMA and their direction. The FDMA flap is designed so that the dorsalis pedis artery and FDMA are at the middle of the flap. It can be extended from the lower margin of extensor retinaculum to the first intermetatarsal area and can be safely raised from the whole width of the foot (Fig. 30.3). A reversed first dorsal metatarsal artery perforator flap measuring 5.0 cm × 3.0 cm was elevated as a pedicle flap (Fig. 30.4).

Flap Elevation

A pneumatic tourniquet is applied and the skin incision is started from the proximal side of the flap so that dorsalis pedis artery is exposed. Dissection is continued distally down to expose the deep planter branch and the FDMA. Care should be taken not to damage the communicating branch between the FDMA and plantar artery. The tourniquet is then released to observe the color of flap. The dorsalis pedis artery and veins in the proximal side of the flap and the deep plantar branch are then clamped for 10 min to ensure that there is adequate circulation. The dorsalis pedis vascular and the deep planter branch are then ligated and divided (Fig. 30.5).

Flap Transfer

The flap was transposed 180° to the defect and the donor site was repaired using a full-thickness skin graft (Fig. 30.6).

Follow-Up

The flap survived smoothly. At 20 days the flap is stable and he is able to wear regular shoes (Fig. 30.7).

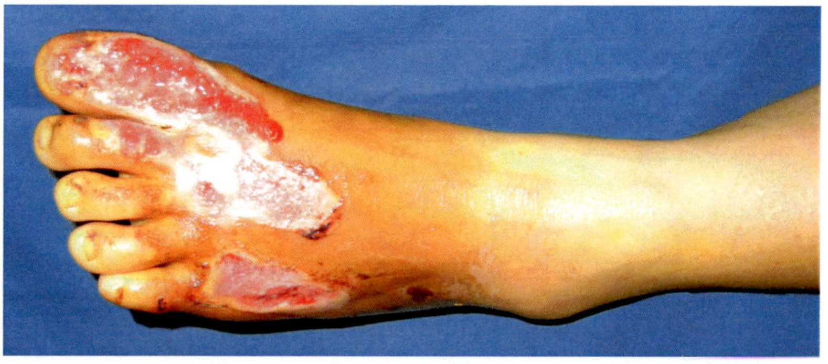

Fig. 30.2 Preoperative view

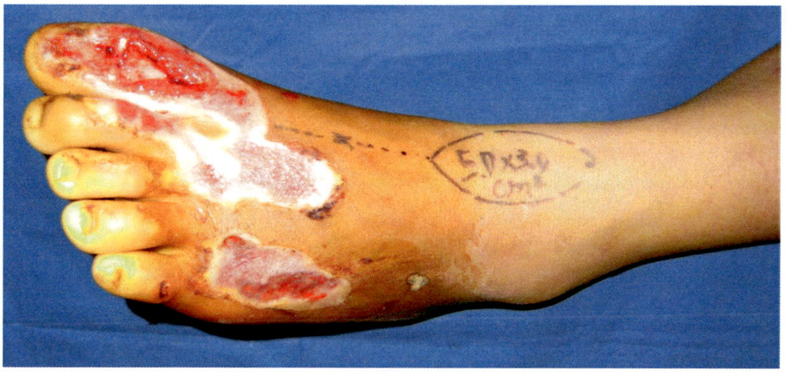

Fig. 30.3 Flap design

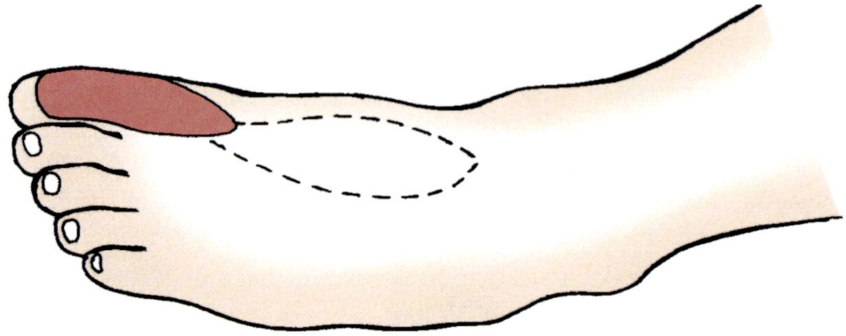

Fig. 30.4 Schematic drawing of flap design

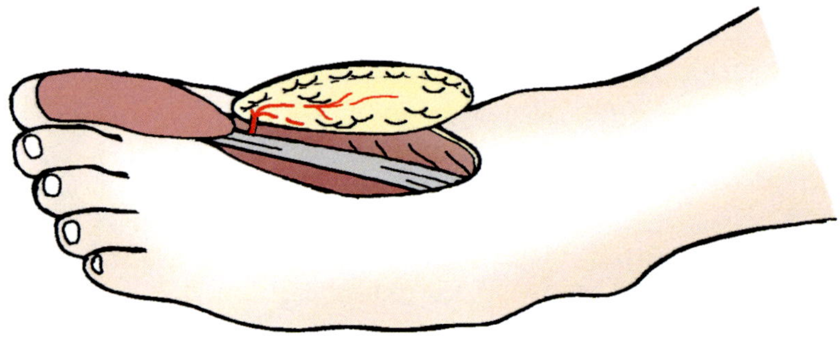

Fig. 30.5 Schematic drawing of the flap elevation

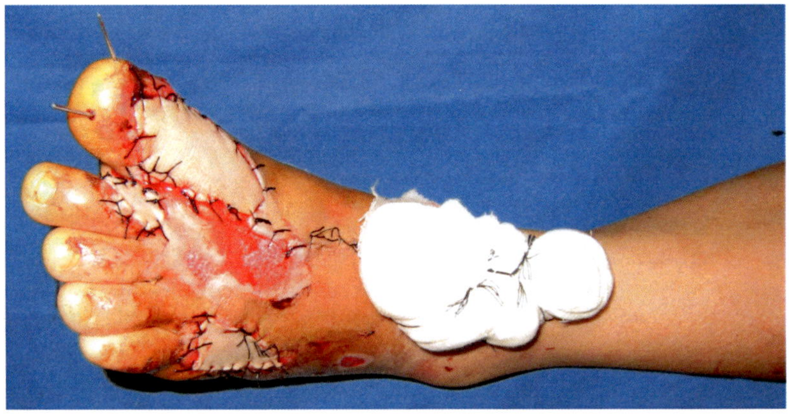

Fig. 30.6 Flap transfer and insetting

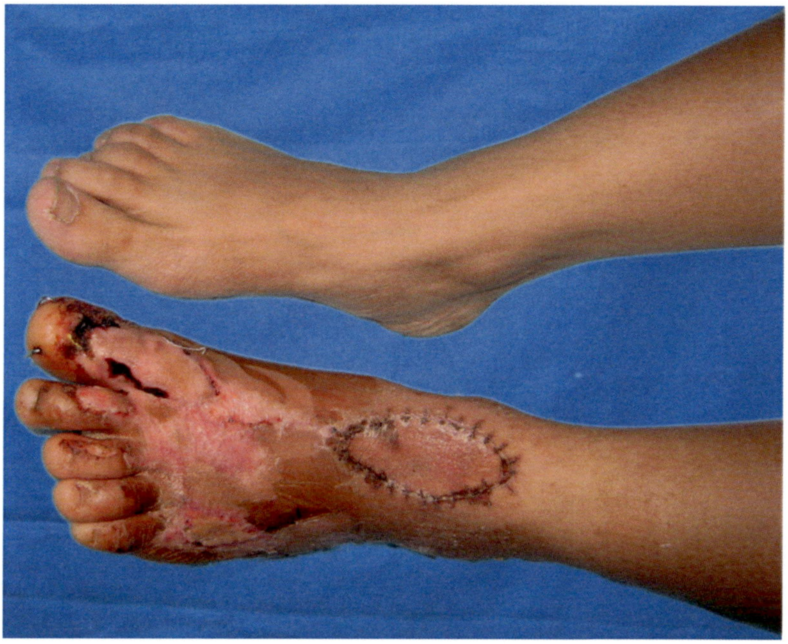

Fig. 30.7 Follow-up

Pearls

The reverse flap, which is based on the FDMA, has along vascular pedicle can be easily transferred to the distal foot [6].

Pitfalls

It should be emphasized that the FDMA is absent in nearly 15 % of cases [3, 7], so preoperative Doppler flowmetry is mandatory to evaluate the dorsalis pedis artery, FDMA, and the communication artery [8, 9].

Before ligating the dorsal artery and vein proximally, the proximal pedicle and deep plantar branch should be clamped for at least 10 min to evaluate the blood inflow and outflow of the FDMA flap. If the blood inflow and outflow of the flap is sufficient, the proximal pedicle is divided and ligated.

To reduce the morbidity of donor site, it is essential and necessary to preserve the peritendon of the exposed tendons on the dorsum of the foot once the flap is elevated.

References

1. Earley MJ, Milner RH. A distally based first web flap in the foot. Br J Plast Surg. 1989;42(5):507–11.
2. Hayashi A, Maruyama Y. Reverse first dorsal metatarsal artery flap for reconstruction of the distal foot. Ann Plast Surg. 1993;31(2):117–22.
3. McCraw JB, Furlow Jr LT. The dorsalis pedis arterialized flap. A clinical study. Plast Reconstruct Surg. 1975;55(2):177–85.
4. Man D, Acland RD. The microarterial anatomy of the dorsalis pedis flap and its clinical applications. Plast Reconstr Surg. 1980;65(4):419–23.
5. Ohmori K, Harii K. Free dorsalis pedis sensory flap to the hand, with microneurovascular anastomoses. Plast Reconstr Surg. 1976;58(5):546–54.
6. Liu L, Cao X, Cai J. Reconstruction of weightbearing forefoot defects with digital artery flaps. J Foot Ankle Surg: Off Publ Am Coll Foot Ankle Surg. 2015;54(1):41–5.
7. Sakai S. A distally based island first dorsal metatarsal artery flap for the coverage of a distal plantar defect. Br J Plast Surg. 1993;46(6):480–2.
8. Pallua N, Di Benedetto G, Berger A. Forefoot reconstruction by reversed island flaps in diabetic patients. Plast Reconstr Surg. 2000;106(4):823–7.
9. Governa M, Barisoni D. Distally based dorsalis pedis island flap for a distal lateral electric burn of the big toe. Burns: J Int Soc Burn Inj. 1996;22(8):641–3.

FSC
www.fsc.org
MIX
Papier | Fördert
gute Waldnutzung
FSC® C083411

Kolibri 360 GmbH
Ferdinand-Jühlke-Straße 7
99095 Erfurt, Deutschland
produktsicherheit@kolibri360.de